Covid-19
New
Normal

Highly Recommended Titles

Crafting an Asian Future in the Post-COVID-19 Asia
edited by Tai Wei Lim
ISBN: 978-981-125-372-0

Impact of COVID-19 on Asian Economies and Policy Responses
edited by Sumit Agarwal, Zhiguo He and Bernard Yeung
ISBN: 978-981-122-937-4

Post-COVID Asia: Deglobalization, Fourth Industrial Revolution, and Sustainable Development
by Hyun-Hoon Lee and Donghyun Park
ISBN: 978-981-122-897-1
ISBN: 978-981-123-023-3 (pbk)

Revitalising ASEAN Economies in a Post-COVID-19 World: Socioeconomic Issues in the New Normal
edited by Hooi Hooi Lean
ISBN: 978-981-122-846-9

Covid-19
New
Normal

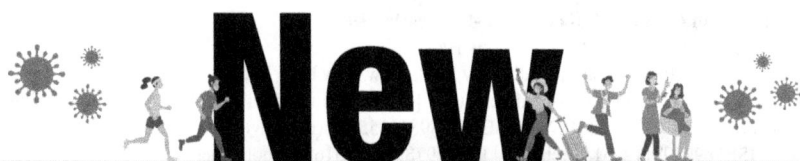
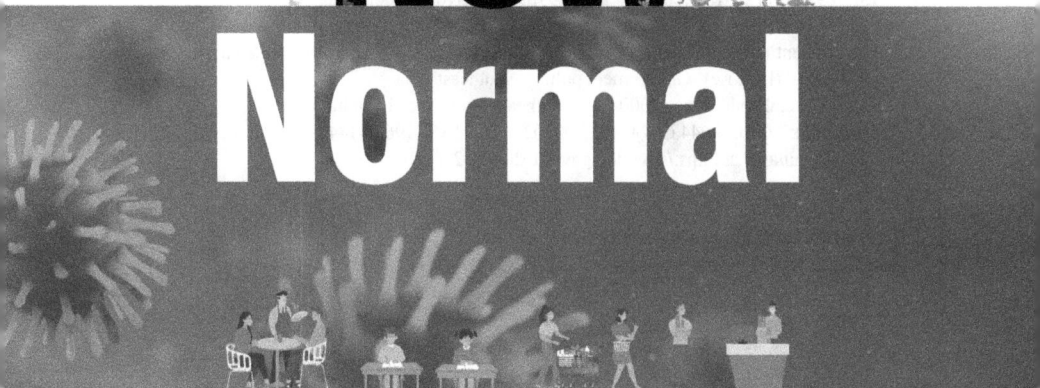

Edited by

Linda LOW
LEE Yew Haur

Singapore University of Social Sciences, Singapore

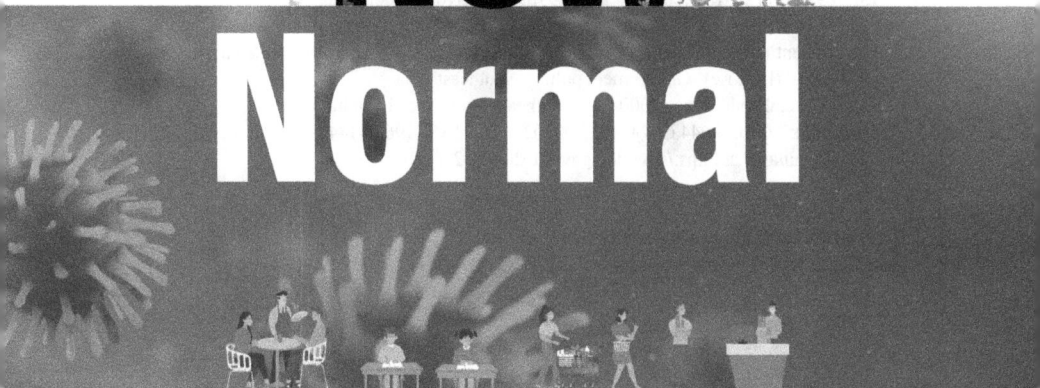 **World Scientific**

NEW JERSEY · LONDON · SINGAPORE · BEIJING · SHANGHAI · HONG KONG · TAIPEI · CHENNAI · TOKYO

Published by

World Scientific Publishing Co. Pte. Ltd.

5 Toh Tuck Link, Singapore 596224

USA office: 27 Warren Street, Suite 401-402, Hackensack, NJ 07601

UK office: 57 Shelton Street, Covent Garden, London WC2H 9HE

Library of Congress Cataloging-in-Publication Data
Names: Low, Linda, editor. | Lee, Yew Haur, editor.
Title: Covid-19 new normal / edited by Linda Low, Yew Haur Lee.
Description: New Jersey : World Scientific, [2023] | Includes bibliographical references and index.
Identifiers: LCCN 2022048782 | ISBN 9789811255144 (hardcover) |
    ISBN 9789811255151 (ebook) | ISBN 9789811255168 (ebook other)
Subjects: LCSH: COVID-19 Pandemic, 2020---Social aspects--China. | COVID-19 (Disease)--
    Government policy--China. | COVID-19 Pandemic, 2020---Social aspects--Southeast Asia. |
    COVID-19 (Disease)--Government policy--Southeast Asia. |
    China--Social conditions--2000– | Southeast Asia--Social conditions.
Classification: LCC RA644.C67 C452258 2023 | DDC 362.1962/41440951--dc23/eng/20221128
LC record available at https://lccn.loc.gov/2022048782

British Library Cataloguing-in-Publication Data
A catalogue record for this book is available from the British Library.

For any available supplementary material, please visit
https://www.worldscientific.com/worldscibooks/10.1142/12802#t=suppl

Desk Editor: Jiang Yulin

Typeset by Stallion Press
Email: enquiries@stallionpress.com

Foreword

The Coronavirus or Covid-19 epidemic that started in 2020 has had an unprecedented impact on society, in terms of its duration, virulence, death toll (in absolute numbers), and certainly in the ways it has conditioned human behavior. A whole new glossary of terms has been invented to describe life during Covid-19, including "lockdown," "safe distancing," "Zoom meeting," "anti-masking," "vaccinated travel lane," "work from home," and of course the "new normal" to which governments, businesses, and individuals are fervently looking forward.

The latter — the future "new normal" that will see the world exit strict Covid-19 restrictions, but with the shadow of another possible epidemic looming over us — is the subject of intense and multifaceted exploration. If the experience of life during Covid-19 was unprecedented, so too is the notion of a life in this liminal state where societies will have to move beyond Covid-19, but in constant readiness for its return.

The present volume assembles a group of scholars to project conditions in China and ASEAN in the new normal. This regional focus is entirely meaningful, given the different challenges facing the different countries in the heterogeneous ASEAN region, and the growing importance of China's influence in this region and the world. The essays touch on crucial topics such as governments' epidemic management, international relations and influences, retail, and related issues of population, health, digitalization, crisis management, various security aspects, and others.

It is of course impossible for any single volume to address all the major issues of the "new normal," but this volume makes a significant contribution to our thinking about this imminent state in the ASEAN and China region. I congratulate the editors and contributors on bringing this edited volume together.

Professor Robbie B. H. Goh
Provost, Singapore University of Social Sciences

About the Contributors

AW Tar Choon is currently Director (Chemical Pathology) at the Department of Laboratory Medicine Changi General Hospital. He holds academic appointments as Clinical Senior Lecturer (Medicine) at the National University of Singapore (NUS) and Clinical Professor (Pathology) at Duke-NUS Graduate Medical School. He has specialist certifications in Internal Medicine (from NUS and the Royal College of Physicians UK) as well as in Chemical Pathology (Royal College of Pathologists of Australasia). He has completed the Harvard–NUS Masters in Public Policy program. He was elected as Fellow of the Royal College of Physicians of Edinburgh (1999), Fellow of the Chapter of Pathologists Academy of Medicine Singapore (2004), and International Fellow of the College of American Pathologists (2020). He has published over 200 journal articles (including 18 on Covid-19) and delivered over 370 lectures in 25 countries (including 12 webinars on Covid-19). He is a recipient of several distinguished national and international awards. He serves on the editorial boards of several journals, including *Nature Scientific Reports.*

CHANG Youngho is Associate Professor and Head of the Business and Management Minors at the School of Business, the Singapore University of Social Sciences (SUSS), Singapore. He specializes in the economics of climate change, economic–energy–environmental modeling, energy and security, oil and macroeconomy, the economics of electricity market deregulation, and green finance and sustainability. He has published more than 70 papers in internationally referred academic journals and edited nine books. He has taught at the National University of Singapore and Nanyang Technological University, Singapore. He received his Ph.D. in Economics (Environmental and Resource Economics) from the University of Hawaii at Manoa, USA.

CHEN Gang is Assistant Director and Senior Research Fellow of the East Asian Institute (EAI), National University of Singapore (NUS). Since he joined the EAI in 2007, he has been tracing China's politics, foreign policy, and environmental and energy policies and publishing extensively on these issues. He is the sole author of *Politics of Renewable Energy in China* (Cheltenham, UK: Edward Elgar, 2019), *The Politics of Disaster Management in China: Institutions, Interest Groups, and Social Participation* (New York: Palgrave Macmillan, 2016), *China's Climate Policy* (London and New York: Routledge, 2012), *Politics of China's Environmental Protection: Problems and Progress* (Singapore: World Scientific, 2009), and *The Kyoto Protocol and International Cooperation against Climate Change* (in Chinese) (Beijing: Xinhua Press, 2008). His research papers have appeared in internationally refereed journals such as *Asian Survey, Asia Pacific Business Review, The Copenhagen Journal of Asian Studies, The International Spectator, The Polar Journal, China: An International Journal, The Chinese Journal of International Politics,* and *The Journal of East Asian Affairs.* He provides consultancy for the Singapore government on policy issues in East Asia. He is frequently interviewed by media like *Bloomberg Television,* the *South China Morning Post, Channel NewsAsia,* and *Xinhua News Agency.* He occasionally gives lectures at NUS.

Allan CHIA is Associate Professor and Dean at the School of Business, Singapore University of Social Sciences. He received his Bachelor of Arts (Hons) at the National University of Singapore and Masters of Commerce in Marketing at the University of Strathclyde, Glasgow.

Gunter DUFEY is Professor Emeritus of Finance, International Business and Strategy at the University of Michigan Ann Arbor, where he joined the faculty after receiving M.A. and Ph.D. degrees from the University of Washington, Foster School in Seattle. He held visiting appointments at Stanford, the University of Texas, and a number of universities in Europe. He concluded his academic career at Nanyang Business School, NTU, in Singapore. He published extensively in the international finance field and had consulting engagements with McKinsey, Monetary Authority of Singapore, and a large number of major financial institutions and multinational corporations.

Carmenchu ECHIVERRI-VILLAVICENCIO is Section Head, Department of Infectious Disease, and Consultant, Department of Medicine, Section of Infectious Disease, at St. Luke's Medical Center, St. Luke's Global City, The Philippines.

KAN Siew Ning is Adjunct Faculty at Singapore Management University and Singapore Institute of Technology. He holds an M.Sc. in Management of Technology from the National University of Singapore. His research interests include knowledge management and technology innovation.

LEE Yew Haur is Associate Professor and Deputy Director in the Business Intelligence and Analytics unit at the Singapore University of Social Sciences. He holds a Ph.D. in Statistics from Virginia Polytechnic Institute and State University, USA. His research interests are in the application of text mining and data mining in education.

Magdeleine LEW Duan Ning is Senior Assistant Director at the Centre for Teaching Excellence at Singapore Management University. She heads the pedagogical practice and education research portfolio at the Centre. Magdeleine also has over a decade of experience as a problem-based learning practitioner. She is also an experienced trainer, having conducted many Continuing Education and Training programs for adult learners (both locally and overseas) in areas relating to classroom facilitation and student assessment in PBL. Magdeleine holds a Ph.D. in Educational Psychology from the Erasmus University Rotterdam, the Netherlands. Her research interests are in the areas of student assessment and learning effectiveness of technology used for teaching.

Linda LOW retired as Associate Professor in the School of Business at Singapore University of Social Sciences at the end of 2021. She holds a Ph.D. in Economics from the University of Singapore, 1984, with books published including a Primer in Economics, Singapore GLCs, Singapore CPF, and others co-authored in the topics of Fintech, Belt and Road Initiative, Covid-19, Economies in Asia Pacific (like China, Japan), Association of Southeast Asian Nations (ASEAN), Gulf Cooperation Council (GCC), etc.

Thomas MENKHOFF is Professor of Organisational Behaviour and Human Resources (Education) at the Lee Kong Chian School of Business, Singapore Management University (SMU). His current research interests center on sustainable innovation at ("smart") city and corporate levels, technology-enhanced learning, and Industry 4.0 adoption by Asian SMEs. One of his latest book publications is *Catalyzing Innovations for a Sustainable Future: Bite-Sized Commentaries and Resource Materials* (World Scientific Publishing, 2021).

Yong POOVORAWAN currently heads the Center of Excellence in Clinical Virology in the Faculty of Medicine at Chulalongkorn University in Bangkok. Professor Poovorawan obtained his M.D. in 1974 from Chulalongkorn University and his specialization in pediatrics in 1978 from Chulalongkorn Hospital and University. In 1984, he was Research Fellow in pediatric hepatology at King's College Hospital Medical School in London. Professor Poovorawan began working in the Department of Pediatrics at Chulalongkorn University as a lecturer and became a full professor in 1991. Professor Poovorawan has received many research awards and honors, including the Outstanding Researcher Award in 1997 from the National Research Council of Thailand, Outstanding Scientist Award in 1997 from the Foundation for the Promotion of Science and Technology under the Patronage of His Majesty the King, Mahidol University-B-Braun Award in 2002, Thailand Research Fund Award in 2004, Outstanding Achievement Doctor from the Medical Council of Thailand in 2018, Achievement Award in Virology, Genetics Society of Thailand in 2018, Achievement Award from the National Vaccine Institute of Thailand in 2019, and Senior Research Scholar by the Thailand Research Fund since 1997. He also received the Outstanding Best Teachers Award in 2004 from the Thailand National University Teacher Association. Competitive grants awarded to him include the Outstanding Professor Thailand Research Fund (2012–2014) and NSTDA Research Chair Grant (2014). He received an outstanding award on vaccine research from the National Vaccine Institute (2020). He is a leading expert in viral hepatitis in Thailand, and from his hepatitis work since 1986, he has contributed to the drastic reduction of hepatitis A, B, and C in Thailand. His research also involves emerging and reemerging viruses, including avian influenza, hand–foot–mouth disease, human papillomavirus, respiratory tract, and enteric diseases. Since the introduction of the Covid-19 into Thailand in 2019, he has led efforts in developing methods to rapidly detect the virus, characterizing virus variants circulating in Thailand, immune response profiles in recovered patients, and immunity induced by vaccination of different vaccines, and has provided consultation of best public health policies to the Thailand government. He currently serves on various committees, including the EPI vaccine, viral hepatitis, and emerging diseases of the Center for Disease Control, Ministry of Public Health. Professor Poovorawan has authored and co-authored more than 640 publications in the fields of vaccine, virology, hepatitis, and pediatric hepatology with H-index 67 on Google Scholar.

Mohan RAVURU is Director of Medical and Scientific Affairs (Asia-Pacific), Abbott Rapid Diagnostics, Singapore.

Karin SIXL-DANIELL is Professor of Management and an entrepreneur and has been a pioneer in online and blended learning, facilitating such courses since 2003. In addition to her being Associate Faculty at the Singapore University of Social Sciences, she has been working in Austria, Canada, the United Arab Emirates, Germany, Hungary, India, Malaysia, and Singapore. She was also Co-Programme Director for the blended Programme on Family Business and Entrepreneurship at the Indian Institute of Management (IIM) in Bangalore. Before focusing on e-learning, Dr. Sixl-Daniell was Assistant Professor and Deputy Head at the Institute of International Management, University of Graz, Austria. She was also a member of the Advisory Panel to the INSEAD Financial Education for Women initiative FinEdX and co-authored the book "Wealth Wisdom for Everyone" which was accompanied by a 26-episode TV series on Channel NewsAsia in 2006. She also established her own research and advisory businesses and holds a Doctorate in Social and Economic Sciences (Business Administration) and two Masters degrees, one in economics and one in healthcare management.

Rontgene M. SOLANTE is Fellow and Diplomate of both the Philippine College of Physicians and the Philippine Society for Microbiology and Infectious Diseases, and Fellow of the Infectious Diseases Society of America (IDSA) and is currently with the San Lazaro Hospital in Santa Cruz, Manila.

Jayarani TAN holds a Ph.D. in Sociology from Universität Bielefeld, Germany, and is Principal Lecturer and Course Coordinator for the course entitled, "Leadership and Teambuilidng SMU-X" at Singapore Management University (SMU). Her research interest is in the use of digital technology in higher education, and she works with an industry partner in the course of her teaching.

Lydia TEO Ying Qian is Research Assistant at Lee Kong Chian School of Business in Singapore Management University. She holds a Bachelor of Social Sciences from Singapore Management University. Her research interests include technology innovation and technology-enhanced learning.

Christopher TOH Meng Sung has gotten the Doctor of Business Administration (DBA) degree from the Singapore University of Social Sciences (SUSS) and a Master of Business Administration (MBA) from Murdoch University. His research interests are in energy and environment sustainability. He has published a commentary on how hydrogen can be viable for Singapore in *The Business Times* of Singapore. Dr. Toh sits on the Singapore Academic Board of Murdoch University in Singapore, representing the interests of students enrolled in its MBA program.

Amy WONG is Associate Professor in the School of Business at the Singapore University of Social Sciences. She holds a Ph.D. in Management from Monash University, Australia. Her research interests include online brand communities, celebrities, and influencers.

Meilin ZHANG is Senior Lecturer in the Business Analytics Program at the Singapore University of Social Sciences, where she has been teaching data analytics, artificial intelligence, business technologies, and digital marketing in the undergraduate, graduate, and executive programs since 2017. Meilin received her B.S. and M.S. degrees in Computer Science from China and her Ph.D. in Decision Science from NUS Business School in 2015. Her research is in the areas of supply chain management, robust optimization, healthcare analytics, sharing economy, large-scale computation, and machine learning. She has also published her work in top-tier business journals *Management Science, Operations Research,* and *Manufacturing & Service Operations Management* (MSOM).

Contents

https://doi.org/10.1142/9789811255151_0001

Chapter 1

Introduction

Linda Low and Lee Yew Haur

Singapore University of Social Sciences, Singapore

Six months after the Omicron variant was first identified by the World Health Organization (WHO) on 24 November 2021, we seem to be seeing the tail end of the spread of Covid-19 Omicron cases while at the same time, the world is now removing travel restrictions and mask wearing is retained only in some settings and/ or regions. At the same time, there is the Russia–Ukraine war that is grinding into its ninth month with no end in sight. As we await news from doctors, scientists, and researchers on either another variant or the eventual demise of Covid-19, it seems that everyone is eager to move on to adjust to the "new normal". Hence, it is timely to have a book on what the "new normal" is like from the economic, political, health, and social perspectives.

Although Covid-19 is a health crisis, the global economy is impacted due to the lockdowns and closure of entire countries to contain the spread of the virus and the subsequent attempts to reopen parts of the economy. And, of course, politics is involved as governments craft policies to govern behavior to contain the virus as well as direct healthcare resources to test, treat, and eventually to eradicate the disease. There is also a social aspect as well, as our leaders and universities have to grapple with how to move forward

1

as it might not be just simply reverting back to what we did in the pre-Covid times.

In quite a few chapters, there has been a focus on China and ASEAN for the following reasons:

(1) China is the rising economic power, as evidenced by the spending power of Chinese tourists in ASEAN as well as in the US and Europe, especially in the luxury goods market. Moreover, China is undoubtedly the factory of the world, as witnessed during the severe global supply chain disruption encountered worldwide when China employed lockdowns to stem the spread of Covid-19 at the start of the pandemic in 2020. Due to the lockdowns, the workers were confined to their homes, and this shuttered the factories producing goods that are consumed worldwide. According to Jie and Wallace [1], China also extended its global reach through the Belt and Road Initiative (BRI) by financing infrastructure projects across Asia, Africa, and Europe in their own currency, the renminbi (RMB), to develop new trade routes connecting China to the rest of the world. Lastly, although Wuhan, China, is the place where the first Covid-19 cases were discovered that eventually spread to the rest of the world, Chinese scientists also contributed to the solution of containing the virus by releasing the genetic sequence of Covid-19 to the world so that researchers worldwide could understand the origin and behavior of the virus [2].

(2) ASEAN, with a population of 675 million, is a regional grouping of 10 countries in Southeast Asia that was originally formed in 1967 during the Cold War to counter the communist threat, among other objectives. Presently, ASEAN is still courted by both the US and China and it will be interesting to examine ASEAN–China relations during Covid-19 to see if ASEAN is still true to the Non-Aligned Movement (NAM) that it was originally part of, which is no longer mentioned. Besides politics, ASEAN is also the food basket of the world in providing food as well as raw materials to support China's role as the factory of the world.

(3) Both China and ASEAN have experience dealing with a similar viral outbreak, i.e., the Severe Acute Respiratory Syndrome (SARS), in 2002. Hence, some comparison is possible, especially in China's crisis management, and this will be done in Chapter 6.

This book is for policymakers, researchers, those in business, and the public interested in how we are adapting to the Covid-19 pandemic from the economic, political, health, and social perspectives.

Beginning with the economic perspective, Chapter 2 looks at the various dimensions of the RMB internationalization in the face of the BRI that uses the RMB for financing. It will be interesting to see if the RMB makes any dent to the dominant position of the USD in the face of China's rising economic clout coupled with the fact that it is the world's largest trading nation and holds the largest reserves of foreign currency.

In Chapter 3, we look at how the global clean energy transition which is driven by climate change has been affected by the Covid-19 pandemic. It also offers a road map for the transition in the post-pandemic era in the ASEAN region that includes green recovery initiatives.

Chapter 4 covers the trends and determinants of the global industrial supply chain and discusses the way forward in the post-pandemic era to overcome the disruption caused to the supply chain.

Another aspect from the economic angle would be the "new normal" in retail, which is covered in Chapter 5. With the initial lockdown in 2020, physical stores were forced to shutter, leading to an increase in online shopping as consumers were forced to stay indoors. This trend has continued even after certain sectors of the economy reopened. Some nimble retailers quickly adapted to this change while others folded during this pandemic. This chapter covers the changing consumer behaviors and the consequent impact on the retail business. Possible post-pandemic retail scenes that have emerged are also covered, with a discussion on the prevalence of new types of retail consumers.

Switching to the political perspective, Chapter 6 looks at how China's crisis management in the handling of the Covid-19 has evolved from that of SARS in 2002, some 18 years apart. The similarities and differences between the handling of the two pandemics are discussed and a mistake that has been repeated is also noted. A timeline of the Chinese government's response to the Covid-19 outbreak between 31 December 2019 and 23 February 2020 is compiled in the Appendix, which might be useful for future researchers in this area.

Chapter 7 looks at ASEAN–China relations spanning from before to during the Covid-19 period and observes that even the former US colony, the Philippines, is having cozy relations with China, as exemplified by the multiple visits that then President Rodrigo Duterte made to China as compared to none being made to the US.

Moving to the health angle, Chapter 8 covers the Covid-19 outlook in ASEAN. The initial containment with lockdowns and travel restrictions, among other measures, in combating the first wave in 2020 is largely successful but the prolonged fight has resulted in fatigue, and the April 2021 wave threatened to overwhelm the healthcare system. The outlook ahead is forecasted and the recommendations with specific mention of testing and vaccination are discussed.

As we learn to cope with Covid-19 as an endemic, the possibility that we might have to face both Covid-19 and influenza as the "twindemic" seems to be a high possibility. Chapter 9 entertains the scenario by first comparing Covid-19 with the Spanish Flu of 1819 and reviewing the timeline and history for the viral disease outbreaks in Asia in the 21st century to provide a historical perspective. The potential public healthcare consequences of having the "twindemic" are discussed, leading to key recommendations to prepare ourselves for this collision course for the region.

From the social point of view, Chapter 10 looks at the "new normal" in teaching and learning with technology in a local university through the reflections and recommendations of several educators to help students stay engaged and focused.

Chapter 11 covers the demand on leaders in the "new normal" as there is more emphasis on work–life balance arising probably from having to work from home while tackling problems like talent shortage.

Lastly, Chapter 12 summarizes the key takeaways from the economic, political, health, and social perspectives that will help us adapt to the Covid-19 "new normal".

References

[1] Jie, Y., and Wallace, J. (2021). What is China's Belt and Road Initiative (BRI)? https://www.chathamhouse.org/2021/09/what-chinas-belt-and-road-initiative-bri.

[2] Schnirring, L. (2020). China release genetic data on new coronavirus, now deadly. https://www.cidrap.umn.edu/news-perspective/2020/01/china-releases-genetic-data-new-coronavirus-now-deadly.

Chapter 2

RMB Internationalization

Gunter Dufey
University of Michigan, USA

1. The Disconnect

1.1 *Introduction*

The last decade has seen significant shifts in the world economy, with a rising Chinese economy challenging that of the US in terms of economic output (GDP) and with China's global reach extending significantly through the Belt and Road Initiative (BRI). The Covid-19 pandemic may have accelerated some of these and related trends. Yet, certain aspects of the international financial architecture have been virtually unchanged. The dominance of the USD in international finance in general, relative to the Renminbi, for short the RMB,[i] has become a recurrent topic, especially during conflicts arising between China and the US. For many years, various US Administrations have used access to its USD payment and financial system to exert pressure on business entities and countries regarding

---

[i] RMB is the term for the Chinese currency, the "people's money." "Yuan" is the term used when reference is made to specific transactions i.e., 1 USD is 6.98 Yuan.

issues it considers as strategic. Indeed, the term "weaponizing the USD" has become a favored expression among commentators.

It is therefore not surprising to note that, with increasing frequency, speculations arise in public discussion and academe about the "internationalization of the RMB." In any case, the internationalization of the Chinese currency is an important topic as it pertains to the emerging role of the People's Republic of China (PRC) in world economics and politics.

The objective of this chapter is to assess the various dimensions of RMB internationalization.

1.2 *Recent developments*

Over the past three decades, China's rapid economic growth and its increasing economic integration with the rest of the world have led to a significant increase in its "weight" in the world economy. China is now arguably the world's largest economy, or about to attain this position by some measures, and it is the largest trading nation. The Chinese government holds the largest amount of foreign exchange reserves in the world. Yet, the international use of the RMB is extremely modest.

As data compiled by the European Central Bank and reproduced in Figure 1 demonstrate, the role of the RMB in international

Snapshot of the international monetary system

(percentages)

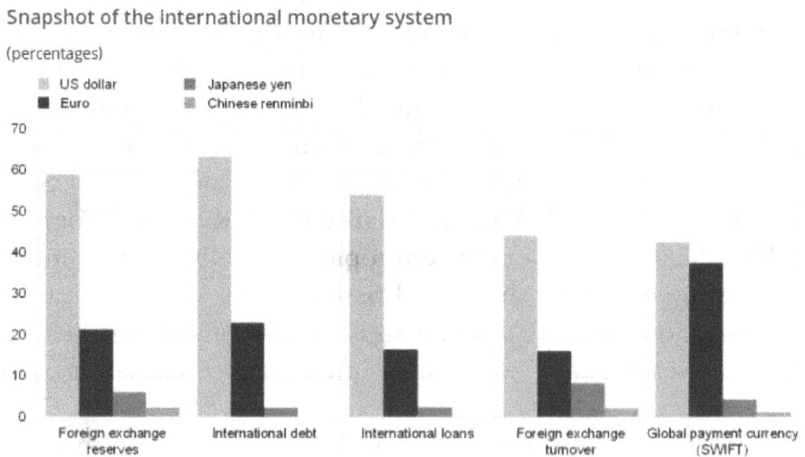

Figure 1. International monetary system (%).

Source: ECB [1].

(left panel: percentages; right panel: index)

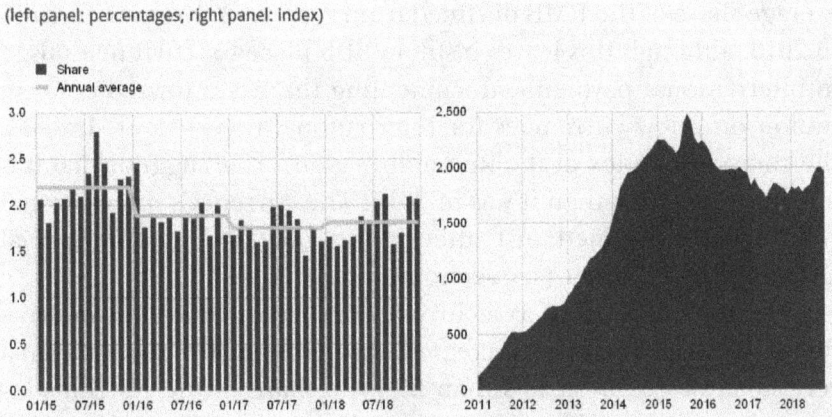

Figure 2. Change in RMB's share as an international payment currency (left panel) and a composite indicator of internationalization (right panel).
Source: ECB [2].

finance remains insignificant, especially in light of the heft that China represents in terms of the "real" economy, as compared to financial markets. Some of that should not come as a surprise. After all, the PRC comprises a huge landmass and contains within it a population of 1.4 billon literate and hard-working people, approximately four times that of the US or the European Union (without Britain).

Nevertheless, there have been some developments. The use of the RMB for international payments has increased. In the two years from 2020 to 2021, its use had grown quite a bit, although from a tiny base, but had seemingly stalled at the time of the writing of this chapter and even decreased slightly, as shown in Figure 2, while the real economy continued to grow at very respectable rates of 5%–6% per year.

One popular indicator of the internationalization of a currency is its role in transborder payments. SWIFT[ii] data show that the

---

[ii] SWIFT or Society for Worldwide Interbank Financial Telecommunication is a cooperative of financial institutions providing a secure and efficient messaging system that conveys settlement (payments) instructions among banks and other large clients, including central banks.

average share of the RMB declined from 2.2% in 2015 to about 1.8% in 2018, although this leaves it still in fifth place for currencies used in international payments, documenting the trend toward concentration on a few currencies for international transactions. Indeed, the composite index of the Renminbi's global role suggests that it is less strong in 2018 than it was in 2015. The currency's international role actually declined just after it was included in the Special Drawing Rights basket (see sections 3.2 and 3.3).

The use of the RMB as a currency of denomination for international bonds and reserves increased noticeably in 2018, again from a very small base. But at less than 2%, the share of the RMB instruments in global foreign reserve portfolios, outstanding amounts of international bonds, and international liabilities remains extremely small overall. However, global central banks' holdings of renminbi-denominated assets in their foreign exchange reserves have increased to a historical high in 2020. A quarterly survey from the International Monetary Fund (IMF) showed that, by the end of March 2020, the share of assets denominated by RMB in global official foreign exchange reserves rose to 2.02%, the highest since the Chinese Yuan was included in the statistics in the fourth quarter of 2016. The determinants of currency denomination of central bank reserve asset will be discussed below. A "Yuan Internationalization Index," released by Renmin University of China, recently summarizes the situation distinctly. While it rose 13% in 2019 to 3.03 and was forecast to rise to 5 in 2020, the currency still trails far behind the USD at 50.85 and Euro at 26.28. By mid-2021, SWIFT data showed the RMB in sixth place, below the CAD, slightly outperforming the AUD.

2. Currency Internationalization

2.1 *Currency fundamentals*

Before the emergence of the medium of exchange, people used to operate an inefficient barter system to obtain goods and services. The next step in the evolution was commodity money. After centuries of commodity-based means of payment[iii] (clam shells, gold,

---

[iii] Actually, paper money was first used during the Tang Dynasty in China.

silver), government-issued "fiat money" has become the prevailing means of payment as, in an ideal world, it can be created at an optimal rate, commensurate with the increase in goods and services (GDP), the ever-present temptation of governments "printing too much" notwithstanding.

Fiat Money depends ultimately on two sets of regulations that buttress currencies:

(1) The respective central bank has been granted a monopoly in creating money, under penalty of law.
(2) The acceptability of a currency is assured by legal tender laws, whereby debt is legally extinguished when the appropriate amount is provided to the creditor at the appropriate time.

However, such laws apply only *within* a country, delineating its jurisdiction. Thus, the use of a national currency outside its home country depends totally on its usefulness for non-residents.

2.2 *What is currency internationalization?*

An international currency is one that is used by non-residents, not merely for transactions with the issuing country's residents but also, and importantly, on occasion for transactions between (third country) non-residents. In other words, an international currency is one that is used instead of the national currencies of the parties directly involved in an international transaction, whether the transaction in question involves a purchase of goods, services, or financial or real assets. The extent of internationalization of a currency is determined by the demand transactors in other countries have for that currency. On an exceptional basis, countries even adopt the currency of another country as their domestic means of payment (see examples below).

Even though the latter phenomenon requires the acquiescence of the local government, essentially, these decisions are made by (private) parties in other jurisdictions; thus, currency internationalization cannot be forced, but must be earned. As an example, when the Government of Ecuador decides to use the

USD as the currency of the realm, this decision comes after private individuals and business firms decided to use USD instead of the local currency.

2.3 *Historical examples*

Monetary history is replete with examples where the currency of another country has replaced in total or in part the local "means of payment." In the US for instance, the Mexican gold Centenario was the preferred means of payment in the South and West of the country when there was no effective central issuing authority, as the Federal Reserve was only established in 1913. By the same token, the British pound was widely used, even outside the British Colonial Empire. More recently, a number of countries have used the USD as their means of payment for domestic transactions, e.g., Panama and Ecuador in South America, Cambodia in Asia, and Liberia in Africa.

2.4 *The vehicle currency concept*

Whenever two parties in different countries enter into a transaction, they must decide in which currency to settle (pay). Except in extreme circumstances, business firms and individuals prefer to do business in their own currency. To accommodate a foreign partner, the purchaser, for example, must have access to the other country's currency, by using the services of a bank that has access to an account in the foreign country, or to maintain his/her own account, if the volume of transactions warrants it.

To maintain such balances is costly and risky, thus there is a strong incentive to minimize foreign balances by concentrating on one currency. Obviously, a currency in which a large volume of transaction is being done has a *prima facie* advantage.

Figure 3 provides an answer regarding the economics of concentrating accounts in one currency (but it does not provide the answer **where** that account is to be held).

Historically, the global payments system has been dominated by a single currency accepted in the exchange of goods and assets among countries. That one currency acts as a "Third-Country-Currency" in the

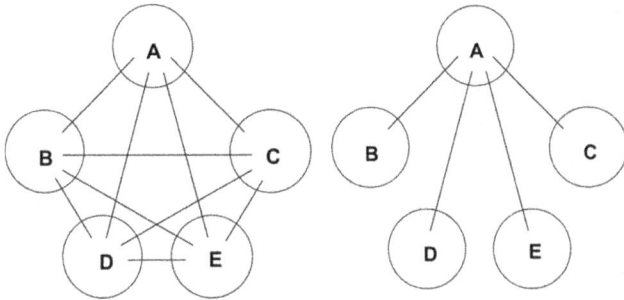

Figure 3. The economics of the vehicle currency.

sense that agents in other economies will generally engage in currency trade indirectly, using the vehicle currency, rather than using direct bilateral exchange among their own currencies. Concentration on one currency saves negotiations on whose currency to use and is efficient as both parties (or their fiscal agents, i.e., banks) maintain settlement accounts in that currency. In addition, the concomitant increase in liquidity makes transactions less costly. To wit, to engage in two related transactions is in the end less burdensome than to act on a bilateral basis.

It is not surprising therefore, that historically the international monetary system has had a predominant currency for facilitating international transactions. Since the middle of the 20th century, the US dollar has played this role. A very large proportion of international exchange in currencies has the US dollar on one side of the transaction. In this sense, the dollar acts as a "vehicle currency."

2.5 *Determinants of vehicle currency competition*

Possessing a large domestic market with a large volume of cross-border trade is the most important criterion for internationalization, as the larger a country's share of world trade and investment, the more likely its currency is to be used by transactors and the more useful is that currency as a unit of account. To wit, after World War I, when the US emerged with a healthy, growing economy, while that of Britain was severely damaged, balances kept by non-residents for international transactions was shifted from London (GBP) to New York (USD).

To some extent, Wall Street, by that time, also surpassed the sophistication of the London financial market. In particular, Wall Street provided extensive "money market" facilities for short-term borrowing and investing, permitting optimal management of liquidity in transaction accounts.

Last but not least, both countries provided a high degree of assurance of *convertibility*,[iv] i.e., the freedom of foreign holders to increase or decrease their balances at will, reflecting the importance of the trust in property rights traditions of these jurisdictions. Therefore, economic size is not the only factor that matters; it may be considered a necessary but not sufficient condition. Indeed, in the context of the internationalization of the RMB, this factor of economic size represents a crucial aspect — yet not the only one as it can be dominated by time zone effects, as will be explained in Section 4.5.

Indeed, "convertibility," or rather the lack thereof, is currently recognized as the major obstacle to the international use of the RMB. Non-residents are very reluctant to entrust their liquid funds to a country that has longstanding policies of limiting the ability of both residents and non-residents to freely increase or decrease balances in their transaction accounts involving cross-border payments. Such "foreign exchange and capital controls" have been an integral part of Chinese economic and financial policy. There is a deeply engrained belief in the political elite of that country that foreign exchange and interest rates are simply too important as levers of control to be left to market forces.

2.6 *Changes in the world economy*

The last few decades have seen significant shifts in the global monetary environment which, in theory, affect one of the determinants of

---

[iv]Convertibility is not an abstract concept relevant for macro-economists, but of real economic significance: the ability to do what you want with your money (as long as its legal), without having to submit a bushel full of papers to ask the relevant authority whether they will permit the payment. For owner of funds abroad, this is a decisive consideration.

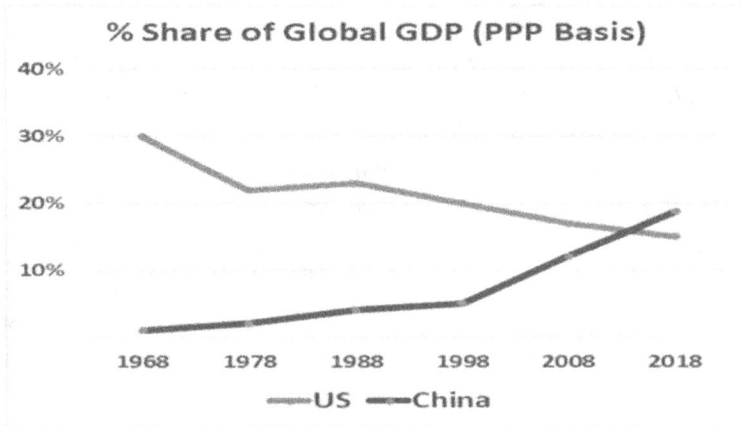

% Share of Global GDP (PPP Basis)

Figure 4. China vs. the US in terms of global GDP.
Source: US Congressional Research.

vehicle currency status. For one, the relative economic size of countries has begun to shift quite significantly during the last four decades as shown in Figure 4. The size advantage of the US has been eroded, simply because the rest of the world, recovering from destructive wars, has significantly offset the relative size advantage of the USD country. First Europe and then Asia (Japan) and, more recently, the PRC, have caught up with the US in terms of economic output. Along with economic size, the associated currencies, in particular the EUR and the Asian "heavyweights," the JPY and more recently the RMB, have come to compete in terms of the underlying dimension of economic size.

Yet, as explained previously, the absolute size of an economy in terms of GDP and its involvement in international trade and investment has only limited impact in light of the agglomeration effect underlying the vehicle currency concept: it is *relative* size that matters, together with related factors explained above.

3. Reserve Currency Status

3.1 *Introduction*

Much of the discussion on "international currency" revolves around the concept of "Reserve Currency." Countries' central banks, in order to influence the value of their currencies in the foreign exchange market, hold reserves in the form of liquid assets denominated in currencies of *other* countries. However, observation quickly shows, they do not just hold liquid assets denominated in *any* foreign currency. Which currencies will they choose?

In postcolonial times, there are no (and never were) international agreements stipulating which currencies are to be chosen; it is a decision that is up to the individual central bank. This decision is influenced by a number of factors, a critical one being the use of that currency in foreign exchange markets. This is because central banks hold foreign monetary assets primarily to influence the foreign exchange value/rate of their own currency relative to others. Thus, there is the phenomenon known as "intervention currency," as ultimately reserves are to be used to "intervene" in the foreign exchange market to affect the exchange rate by buying and selling the domestic for a foreign currency. Since foreign exchange transactions are largely undertaken by private traders and investors, including speculators and "market makers" in financial institutions, the major determinant of central bank holdings is the private market, as this is where the central bank needs to intervene by buying and selling, if they do not like the market rate. Thus, there is a direct link to the vehicle currency, although political and diversification considerations may play a modest role in the allocation process.[v]

3.2 *The RMB as reserve currency*

As far as the share of the RMB in global official holdings of foreign exchange reserves is concerned, it increased in 2019 from a very small base. At constant exchange rates, the share of the RMB in globally disclosed holdings of foreign exchange reserves rose by more than a full percentage point between the end of 2017 and the end of 2019. The share of global foreign reserves held in RMB stood

---

[v]The drivers of denominating "official reserves" differ from those denominating so-called Sovereign Wealth Funds, where some countries accumulate "reserves for a rainy day." Since daily liquidity is secondary, considerations of general portfolio management apply, i.e., risk and return, including diversification, over a longer-term horizon, which includes consideration of currency denomination.

toward the end of 2019 at 2.01%, equivalent to US$219.6 billion. As of the end of 2020, the currency accounted for 2.25% of global foreign exchange assets, an increase of 14.8% year-on-year; as with the presence of extensive data in an emerging economy like China, this shows impressive growth rates on small bases.

China, the world's second-largest and a rapidly developing economy, issuing a "reserve currency" is something that China's leaders find attractive. Along these lines, in recent years, a number of countries acquired modest amounts of RMB bonds for inclusion in their reserve assets. Most recently, Australia joined a small but growing band of central banks that have looked to China for diversification of their foreign reserves. Chile, Japan, and Malaysia are among those holding some RMB assets in their official reserves, while Nigeria's central bank holds around 10% of its reserves in assets denominated in the Chinese currency. Moreover, Japan became the first major developed country to receive approval to invest directly in Chinese sovereign debt. The numbers remain small, however. Governments, like private investors, will continue to be reluctant to invest in assets in a currency that is non-convertible, that is, they are not free to exchange it for other currencies, goods and services, or assets at will. Figures 5 and 6 provide information about the composition of reserve assets held by central monetary institutions.

Over the last few years, a number of countries have concluded so-called *swap lines* with the People's Bank of China (PBoC), just like they have with the US Federal Reserve for a long time. Under these arrangements, countries can quasi-automatically borrow RMB against their own currencies, to be repaid at the original exchange rate after a relatively short period. However, there are no reports that these swap lines have actually been used. In particular, credit facilities under the so-called Chiang Mai Initiative, concluded in 2000 after the Asian Financial Crisis and subsequently expanded in 2012, have never been used.

When everything is said and done, the US dollar still commands by far the largest share of such official holdings. While that figure dropped from 66% in 2014 to approximately 60% at the end of 2020, this drop simply reflected a global tendency toward diversifying

Developments in the shares of the euro, US dollar and other currencies in global official holdings of foreign exchange reserves

(percentages; at constant Q4 2019 exchange rates)

- Euro (right-hand scale)
- US dollar (left-hand scale)
- Other currencies (right-hand scale)

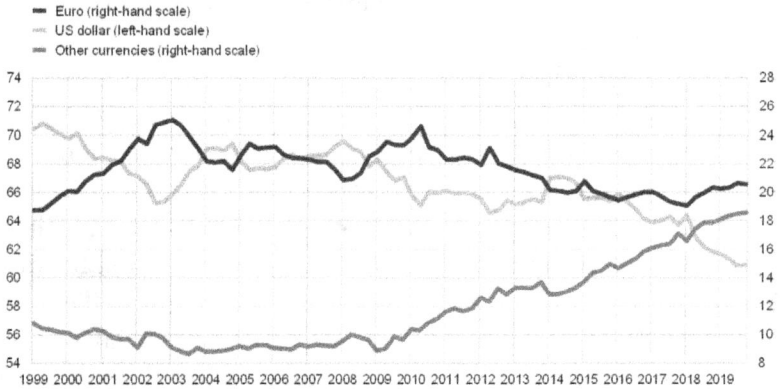

Figure 5. Global official holdings of foreign exchange reserves.

Source: ECB [3].

(percentages; at constant Q4 2019 exchange rates)

- Japanese yen
- Australian dollar
- Pound sterling
- Canadian dollar
- Chinese renminbi

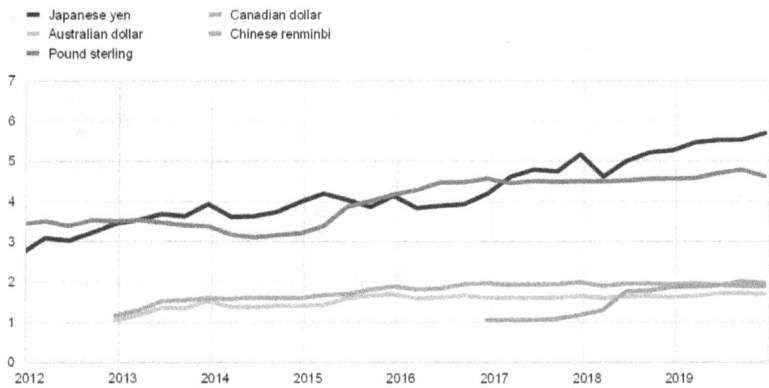

Figure 6. Development in the share of selected currencies in global official holdings of foreign exchange reserves.

Source: ECB [3].

foreign reserves and shifting to currencies of emerging markets. The rising status of the RMB as a reserve currency represents in part the tendency by central banks to diversify holdings of foreign exchange reserves, and in part the growing economic and political influence of China through endeavors such as the BRI. Yet, this recognition of the RMB should not be overestimated: even the bulk of the debt incurred in these transactions is largely denominated in USD.

At this point, the real innovation of RMB internationalization has been the establishment of the **RMB offshore market**, explained in Section 4.4.

3.3 *Expanding the Special Drawing Rights*

The IMF, created as a "cooperative" for member countries in the waning days of World War II, assists members with credit facilities and policy advice during periods when they call for assistance as they are about to default on their international financial obligations. While funded by member contributions, largely based on countries' size and participation in international trade, in 1969, the IMF supplemented its resources with the creation of Special Drawing Rights (SDRs), essentially special "fiat money," whose value reflects a basket of four currencies — the USD, the EUR, the JPY, and the GBP — whose value is determined by weights of 42%, 37%, 11%, and 9%, respectively.

In November 2015, the RMB joined the SDR basket in addition to the previously included four currencies. The RMB was given a weight of approximately 15%, depending on foreign exchange values, with the weight of the other currencies reduced accordingly. It turned out that the inclusion of the RMB in the SDR basket had very little consequences for real economic transactions. The SDR remains purely an accounting currency internal to the IMF, but satisfies China's request to "internationalize" its currency and be recognized, befitting it size and stature in the world economy. Indeed, since voting rights in the IMF are allocated according to weight of a country's contribution, China's voice became stronger.

4. China's Motivations

4.1 *Introduction*

Due to the 2008–2009 Global Financial Crisis, the Chinese government began to promote RMB internationalization in order to raise
its international status, to decrease its reliance on the USD, and possibly to advance domestic financial market reform. An "international
RMB" would spur growth and increase in sophistication of the financial sector and make domestic banking institutions more competitive
internationally. Another motivation for some in China is the liberalization of internal financial markets. Liberalization includes
eliminating restrictions such as bank interest rate ceilings; reserve
requirements; barriers to entry, particularly foreign financial intermediaries; and credit allocation decisions. Such liberalization
reduces the government's interference in financial markets, leading
to the privatization of state-owned banks, improvement of pruden-
tial regulation, and promotion of local stock markets. The necessity
of such policies is documented by the growth of a very large "shadow
banking" sector in China, which led to the emergence of not only
leading payment technologies (e.g., ANT, WeChat Pay) but also
many instances of abuse of such systems.

Apart from prestige and geopolitical considerations, what are
the pros and cons of currency internationalization?

4.2 *Benefits of international currency status*

Looking at this issue from a US perspective, the first benefit is the
"Seigniorage Revenue." Seigniorage may be counted as revenue for
a government when the money it creates is worth more than it costs
to produce it. This revenue is used by governments to finance por-
tions of their expenditures without having to collect taxes. It is
estimated to generate in some years over US\$10 billion for the US
Treasury.

The second benefit is that the US can raise capital more cheaply
due to large purchases of US Treasury securities by foreign governments and government agencies. McKinsey estimates that these

purchases reduced the US borrowing rate by 50 to 60 basis points in recent years, generating a financial benefit of US$90 billion.

The role of an international currency gives a country both economic and political power. The recent settlement between the French BNP and the US Government regarding violation of US sanctions on Iran would not be possible had the US not used the threat of possibly excluding the bank from using the USD payment system for international transactions.

There are broader benefits that are associated with currency internationalization, which was demonstrated in the discussion of the determinants of vehicle currency: it is closely associated with the quality of financial markets in general. Thus, private individuals from all over the world will diversify a portion of their savings in financial assets (bonds, equities, etc.) issued in the country. Moreover, in a world of economic growth, there are ever more savers who look for a safe haven with strong property rights and institutions that protect the rights of investors. Of course, from an accounting perspective, such capital inflows show up as "balance of payment deficits," but those are clearly of a different nature than the deficits that countries incur to finance growing investments or, more problematically, excess consumption. While it is not always easy to distinguish between "good" or "bad" deficits, the currency of denomination of debt-contracts in local or foreign currency is a useful first indicator. Countries whose balance of payments deficits are considered "bad" will not be able to sell debt instruments denominated in their national currency abroad.

4.3 *Disadvantages of internationalization*

Internationalization of a currency does not come without costs and risks. The steady demand of foreigners for liquid assets in the currency drives up its value (exchange rate), causing pain to export industries, fostering imports, and hurting import-competing industries. While the overall supply of good and services increases, significant sectors, including labor, may be hurt.

Amidst such change, financial systems become subject to external shocks ("macro-economic instability"). In particular, there is "settlement risk" for local financial institutions when foreign counterparties default, with concomitant potential risk to taxpayers.

It is not surprising therefore that small countries, such as Switzerland and Singapore, have actively and successfully discouraged the international use of their currencies. Yet, while it is quite easy to prevent internationalization of a currency (by curtailing external convertibility), it is very difficult to attain it as it is transactors in other countries that decide on the international use of a currency.

4.4 *Growth of an offshore market for RMB deposits*

The real innovation at this point of RMB internationalization has been the establishment of the RMB offshore market, allowing financial institutions outside of China to offer RMB liabilities (deposits) and create RMB assets, i.e., loans and fixed income securities, similar to a market that evolved in the mid-1960s, involving major convertible currencies, primarily the USD, and generating a special set of interest rates, known as LIBOR, currently replaced by other indices.

Given China's interest in promoting an international role for the RMB, for reasons of prestige and possibly hope in some quarters that this would ultimately lead to a liberalization of the domestic financial market, the establishment of an offshore market began in 2003. Offshore use of the RMB expanded rapidly in Hong Kong SAR as China sought to develop an international role for its currency, while maintaining strict capital controls. Banks in Hong Kong were permitted and even encouraged to accommodate the demand for RMB deposits and other liquid investments by non-residents during a period that was characterized by a steady rise of the value of the RMB in foreign exchange markets, as suggested in Figure 7.

Conditions for the existence and growth of an offshore market for intermediated funds are first and foremost that external financial intermediaries, so-called "offshore banks" that accept (savings-)

Renminbi per dollar

China kept the renminbi little
_ changed against the dollar
during the global financial
crisis.

6.957

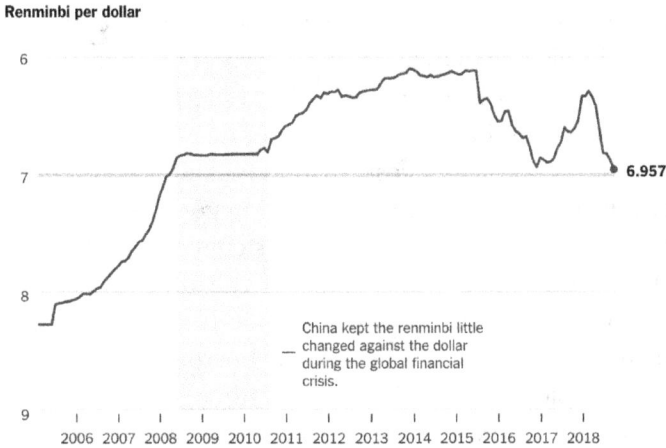

Figure 7. RMB vs. USD forex rates.

Source: Bloomberg.

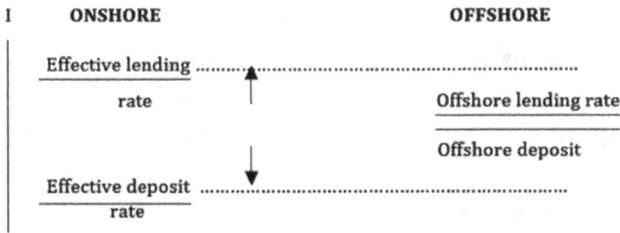

| ONSHORE | OFFSHORE |

Effective lending rate

Offshore lending rate

Offshore deposit

Effective deposit rate

Figure 8. Offshore/Onshore interest rates.

Source: Dufey and Giddy [4].

deposits denominated in other than the local legal tender, must have sufficient cost advantages to overcome the risk perceptions of depositors by paying higher interest rates than available in the respective national market. Thus, effective USD interest rates on dollar deposits in London (LIBOR based) must be higher than equivalent rates in New York. By the same token, the offshore banks must be able to provide lower cost credit facilities than are available in the US domestic market. Figure 8 illustrates these conditions. They are able to do so because the cost of intermediating funds outside the country where a (convertible) currency is means of payment is simply due to the fact that the cost of taking (time-) deposits and making loans is less than in the respective domestic market. The reasons are found on the avoidance of mandatory reserve requirements and other regulatory costs such as making less profitable loans to politically preferred customers, including government entities.

As far as the RMB offshore market is concerned, the economics are slightly different: the advantage of the offshore banks was to offer non-residents RMB deposits, something that exchange controls did not permit in the PRC. Yuan borrowers required special permits to deploy the funds within China. Politically important Chinese entities and select foreign investors received such permissions, advantageous because the cost of funds turned out to be less that the alternatives available within the PRC.

Of course, when the volumes of settlements for deposits and loans differ on a given day, the offshore banks must have unrestricted access to the payment system in the country where the currency is means of payment. This is why there are no offshore markets for important currencies like the Indian Rupee (INR) and the Singapore Dollar (SGD) where non-resident convertibility is limited [4].

However, these offshore deposits cannot be used for payments, like domestic (demand-) deposits. The offshore banks can use deposits and offset them only against offshore out-payments. Any discrepancy must be settled via the national payment system of the currency in question on the books of the respective Central Bank. This is why convertibility matters. As far as the RMB is concerned, the PBoC got around this fundamental problem by instituting a system of "clearing banks" — first was Bank of China HKG, and subsequently other Chinese state banks in other major countries — to settle RMB payments originating in the offshore market. Figure 9 illustrates the clearing of offshore RMB deposits in Hong Kong. These financial institutions have access to the clearing facilities of the PBoC in Beijing to settle differences in daily inflows and outflows — albeit to a limited extent, evidenced by the emergence of an exchange rate, known as CNH that differs

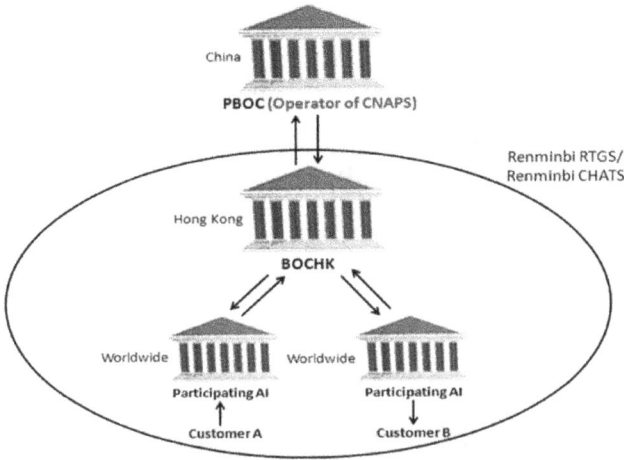

Figure 9. Illustration of Renminbi clearing in Hong Kong.

Source: Anonymous working paper.

from the official exchange rate set by the PBoC inside China for approved international transactions, known as CNY. Interestingly, such differences exist for no other currency used in the offshore market since access to national settlement facilities is readily available, which is the essence of convertibility.

This ingenious system "squared the circle" by providing a degree of "internationalization" of the RMB, without abandoning the system of strict capital and settlement controls governing inflows and outflows of funds from China, in spite of unavoidable leakages between the two markets. Of course, for that market to prosper and grow, non-residents who, because of capital controls, do not have access to deposit facilities in China, must find RMB liquid balances attractive. That attraction wanes when expectations about RMB appreciation fade. This is why data suggest the offshore market for RMB deposits has shrunk at times.

Greater volatility is more likely to be seen in the CNH than the CNY when they respond to the same event. For instance, from May 2018 to August 2018, both the USD/CNH and the USD/CNY rose from a 15-month low to high, largely driven by the US–China trade

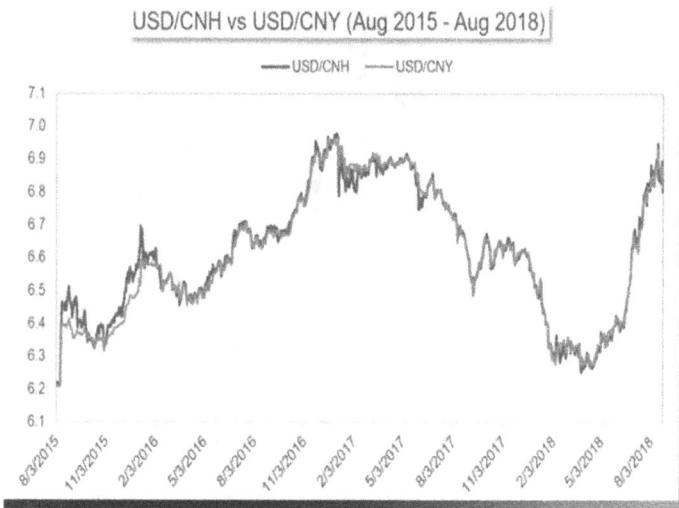

Figure 10.   CNY/CNH vs. the USD.

Source: Bloomberg.

war. The USD/CNH advanced from 6.2358 to 6.9587 while the USD/CNY increased from 6.2419 to 6.9347. Credible reports confirm that PBoC intervention keeps such discrepancies small, as shown in Figure 10.

4.5 *Time-zone effects and the emergence of a CBDC*[vi]

In foreign exchange markets, it is of course possible to obtain a price, known as the "forward price," any time of the day, but final settlement is only possible during Central Bank operating hours in the respective country.

For managers of liquidity, time zones are important, as unexpected in- and out-payments occur frequently, resulting in too much or too little money in their respective transaction accounts. Too much money involves opportunity losses for funds that are part of

---

[vi] Central Bank Digital Currency, sometimes referred to as DC/EP Digital Currency/Electronic Payment.

Table 1. Comparing closing time for central bank settlement.

Country	Central Bank Settlement Closing Time (Local Time)
FED	6:30 p.m. ET (6:30 p.m.)
	The Fedwire Funds Service operates actually 21.5 hours each business day, from 9:00 p.m. NY time on the preceding calendar day to 6:30 p.m. Offline participants can initiate payments or other requests from 9:00 a.m. to 6:00 p.m.
CHIPS	5:00 p.m. ET (5:00 p.m.)
ECB	6:00 p.m. CET (12 noon US)
PoBC (CIPS)	5:00 p.m. CST (5:00 a.m.)*

*US next day during summertime, winter 6:00 a.m.

the total resources of a business, to be short involves incurring penalty interest and reputational damage. Having more time in running a transaction account at the end of the business day makes it easier to manage what is commonly referred to as an "inventory optimization" problem under uncertainty. Thus, a currency that has longer business hours at the end of a given business day is more useful for persons and business entities making cross-border transactions, everything else the same (Table 1).

For that reason, financial managers throughout the world are very much aware of bank cut-off times for settling transactions in various currencies, which in turn are dependent on cut-off times of the respective central bank on whose books "final" clearing takes place as only the central bank has sufficient funds in the local currency so that liquidity, i.e., availability of funds, is never an issue.

The historical fact[vii] that the dateline runs over the Pacific creates special challenges for the international role of Asian currencies in general. To wit, the JPY never attained a significant role, in spite of the fact that it is supported by a large and sophisticated economy,

---

[vii]The origins of the international dateline running through the middle of the Pacific are shrouded in mystery. Myths trace the origin back to Pope Gregory XIII, adjudicating a conflict between Spain and Portugal about their Asian expeditions where one reached sailing around Africa and the other via the Americas, meeting in Asia at the same time on different days. Ultimately, an international conference in 1884 discussed the details but avoided an ultimate conclusion.

with a financial system to match, that was number two for many years, whose business entities are very active internationally and who has adopted convertibility in the early 1980s already.

The key to making RMB more attractive relative to other currencies would be to offset the time-zone effect. Since USD settlement currently is available until 5:00 PM NY time via CHIPS, or 6.00 PM for the "Fedwire" system, for the RMB to equalize, PBoC clearing would have to be available until 5:00 AM or 6.00 AM (summer time) **the next day**.

Could technology bring change when it comes to time-zone constraints? In this context, the creation of so-called CBDC is frequently mentioned, and reliable reports suggest that China is a leader in this field. A digital currency is legal tender, created by the country's central bank. Unlike in a traditional financial system, where only licensed banks have accounts for final settlement with the central bank, here firms and individuals have accounts with the central bank itself, or its special processing entity. The accounts will be linked to the account holder's smartphone number, with transactions taking place through an app, and users can transfer money directly between accounts by tapping phones. This is how digital currency accounts will differ from "digitized deposits" in commercial banks, which will now be bypassed by CBDC.

There is no doubt that digital currencies have the potential to bring about significant changes in the financial system of countries. For example, if widely used, a country's liquid funds will now be concentrated in the Central Bank which — unless it wants to enter the lending business — must subsequently allocate the funds to the commercial banking sector for lending. Without doubt, there will be an advance in the efficiency of the payment system. For the better or worse, the government will have total insight into the financial activities of what individuals and organizations do with their money, probably a very attractive aspect for China, much less so in societies of the West, where people are concerned about privacy.[viii]

[viii] Of course, even in a traditional banking system, the authorities have the ability to trace payments through the banking system, but this is much more cumbersome and in many countries requires court-orders and other impediments. Only cash payments and detours via cryptocurrencies like bitcoin provide privacy.

Nevertheless, as far as internationalization is concerned, CBDC will provide quite limited advances. For one, it is possible to reduce the factor of Central Bank cut-off time. Theoretically it is possible to extend clearing hours to just before midnight Beijing time. Still, the extension of payment times of six or seven hours may be of some tangible value, but mainly to regional players.

By the same token, the effect on the crucial aspect of *convertibility*, and therefore internationalization, is difficult to assess. While it may offer the authorities the ability to fine-tune permissible transactions by account holder (residents vs. non-residents), leakages cannot be avoided, which will frustrate the whole purpose of exchange and capital controls to begin with.

5. Summary and Outlook

Beneath the discussion about the internationalization is a discrepancy. Economic theory of agglomeration and historical experience suggest strongly that the currency of a large trading nation will play a significant role in the international financial system. Yet, the RMB's role in international finance is certainly underwhelming compared to China's weight in the "real" (non-financial) world economy. China accounts for 15.5% of world GDP in nominal financial terms and considerably more in purchasing power terms (vs. 23.6% for the US), almost 15% of merchandise trade (vs. 12% for the US), and 10% of outward foreign direct investment (vs. 20% for the US). But the RMB's share of central banks foreign exchange reserves, 3 years after it became a component of the SDR at the IMF, is only around 2%, compared to 60% for the US dollar, 20% for the Euro, and around 5% each for the Japanese yen and British pound.

The crucial point in assessing the use of a national currency for international transactions is ultimately a matter of assessing the *relative preferences* of entities who buy and sell goods and services across and/or undertake investments (which are simply *future* goods and services).

In this context, it is important to emphasize again that the international use of a currency is decided by transactors *outside the country* where the currency is means of payment, and by this measure China, or any other country, has very little influence. Even bilateral transactions require the consent of the non-Chinese party to accept Yuan, resulting so far in less than 30% of China's own exports and imports being denominated in its home currency in spite of Chinese government policies promoting the use of the Yuan to invoice trade transactions. Clearly, people in other countries have an aversion to using the RMB for payments and investments and currently a corresponding strong preference for using the USD (and to a lesser extent the EUR).

What explains this anomaly? The most important reason is the Chinese government's strong need to control its financial system, including the currency, which injects what are often opaque politics into the determination of its value, and introduces concerns about property rights. The government controls international transactions in RMB for both residents and non-residents. This means in practice that foreigners cannot hold money balances in China without special permission, which can and has been withdrawn at any time. Such a regulatory regime is referred to as "convertibility" — the freedom to obtain and spend Yuan — and in China that freedom has always been lacking, for both residents and non-residents.

Establishing convertibility and the development of trust over the longer term in "property rights" and the concomitant "rule of law" will take decades. To set this process in motion alone will require deep-seated changes in the Chinese economy and financial market, as external financial transactions cannot effectively be separated from domestic markets. To leave crucial decisions about interest and exchange rates and ultimately the allocation of capital to uncontrollable market forces will require figuratively speaking, and possibly literally, a revolution of the political system. While some observers may hope for such changes, very few predict this to happen within a reasonable time horizon. The Chinese political system has proven its resilience against liberalization reforms initiated at home and from abroad.

Even in terms of size-advantage, it is necessary to recognize that Chinese economic growth will continue, but is bound to slow down.

Population dynamics are not propitious. Urbanization has largely run its course, and birth rates have been falling and will go down further. Improving an underfunded healthcare system for a rapidly aging population and dealing with environmental degradation will consume enormous resources. The system of benefiting from comparative advantage through international trade is threatened by conflicts and political "de-globalization."

In the end, lingering effects of convertibility and time-zone disadvantages will frustrate RMB internationalization. Under the very best of circumstances, one might see an emerging role of the RMB in transactions within Asia, where trade and investment links are destined to grow. Comparisons with the JPY might provide a useful start to assess the future. In spite of 40+ years history of free convertibility and a large economy that is well integrated into the world economy via trade and direct investment, the JPY plays a distinctly distant role, way behind the EUR and the USD.

From our analysis, the RMB obviously has the advantage of being the currency of a very large economic entity with a huge international trade and investment sector. To achieve internationalization, capital and money markets in the home country must be not only open and free of controls but also deep and well-developed, with a history of assured property rights. The example of Japan is illustrative in this context.

References

[1] ECB. (2021). The international role of the euro. Retrieved from: https://www.ecb.europa.eu/pub/ire/html/ecb.ire202106~a058f84c61.en.html#toc4. Accessed on 21 November 2022.

[2] ECB. (2019). The international role of the euro. Retrieved from: https://www.ecb.europa.eu/pub/ire/html/ecb.ire201906~f0da2b823e.en.html. Accessed on 21 November 2022.

[3] ECB. (2020). The international role of the euro. Retrieved from https://www.ecb.europa.eu/pub/ire/html/ecb.ire202006~81495c263a.en.html. Accessed on 21 November 2022.

[4] Dufey and Giddy, The International Money Market, Prentice Hall 1994.

https://doi.org/10.1142/9789811255151_0003

Chapter 3

Pandemic and Energy Transition: Perspectives on the New Normal in the Energy Sector in the ASEAN Region

Chang Youngho and Christopher Toh Meng Sung

Singapore University of Social Sciences, Singapore

1. Introduction

The world has had its fair share of unprecedented crises of which the Covid-19 pandemic has had an unanticipated impact on energy transition in the 21st century. The impact from the Covid-19 pandemic has been multi-dimensional across different businesses and industries and for the energy sector, there has been extreme volatility in energy prices, ranging from the continued downturn in the energy market in the first half of 2020 to a drastic antithesis where energy prices have jumped to a record high of more than US$100 a barrel presently. The pandemic has also led to a disrupted global energy supply chain and the plunging fossil fuel prices have also weakened the price competitiveness of renewable energy. Although these negative effects have impeded the energy transition, more voices are calling for a quicker transition to a low-carbon world. The increased risk of fossil fuel investment and the unique advantages of renewable energy demonstrated during the pandemic will create new opportunities for energy transition.

Many countries have been proposing and implementing a variety of strategies in order to achieve green recovery, energy efficiency, and transition post the pandemic. This chapter provides a comprehensive review of the dynamics between global energy transition and the Covid-19 pandemic. The post-pandemic period is a critical time for energy transition around the world. An effective recovery plan shall promote economic recovery without compromising the efforts of global energy transition. Therefore, an effective integration of a "green plan" in the economic recovery scheme is highly recommended in the post-Covid-19 era. Using energy data from the International Energy Agency [1], we first summarized and reviewed the progress of energy transition prior to, during, and post Covid-19. Building on this progression, we will also identify the challenges for energy transition during the pandemic and post the pandemic from the perspectives of government support, fossil fuel divestment, renewable energy production capacity, global supply chain, and energy poverty. However, the pandemic also generates opportunities for global energy transition. We hence also identified potential opportunities for energy transition presented by the pandemic from the perspectives of price competitiveness, policy implementation efficiency, and renewable energy strengths.

The structure of the chapter is as follows. Section 2 looks at some of the more significant energy crises to date, while Section 3 reviews how the present Covid-19 pandemic has shaped the demand and supply of energy. Section 4 discusses the implications for energy demand and supply in a post-pandemic era. Section 5 concludes this chapter.

2. Energy Crises in the World

In the last century, the world has seen some very significant economic depressions such as the Wall Street Crash of 1929, followed by the Great Depression which lasted till 1933. This was immediately followed by the Recession of 1937–1938, which is sometimes called "the recession within the depression" as it came at a time when the recovery from the Great Depression was far from complete and the unemployment rate was still very high. Some scholars have attributed the Recession of 1937–1938 to both monetary and fiscal contractionary policies which worked to reduce aggregate demand, whereas their basis of argument is that it is relevant to today's situation of the Covid-19 pandemic because it illustrates the dangers of a premature withdrawal of stimulus when the economy is still weak [2,3].

As mentioned earlier, the next crisis in the last century was the 1973–1975 recession where there was a period of economic stagnation, high unemployment, and high inflation in much of the Western world during the 1970s, putting an end to the overall post-World War II economic expansion. Among the causes was the 1973 oil crisis. This 1973 oil shock is one of the five critical energy crises that have radically changed the views about energy — with regard to how a major energy crisis can cause rising prices for groceries, car, rent, and just about everything else [4]. The 1970s' energy crisis occurred when the Western world, particularly the United States (U.S.), Canada, Western Europe, Australia, and New Zealand, faced substantial petroleum shortages as well as elevated prices. The oil crisis of the 1970s was brought about by two specific events occurring in the Middle East, the Yom-Kippur War of 1973 which led to price increases and the Iranian Revolution of 1979 which led to supply issues [5]. Both events resulted in disruptions of oil supplies from the region which created difficulties for the nations that relied on energy exports from the region. This oil crisis that happened almost 50 years ago, where the Americans suffered from what contemporaries called "the energy crisis", is a crisis which in many ways shaped the decade of the 1970s. During the twin oil shocks of 1973 and 1979, oil supplies dropped and prices soared, and this resulted in a panic at the pump, fearing there is not enough oil to fill up the gas tanks, heat up homes, or run factory productions [5].

Following the twin oil shocks of the 1970s, the second critical incident was the 1980s' oil glut which was a serious surplus of crude oil caused by falling demand following the 1970s' energy crisis.

During 1979–1980 period, crude oil prices were rapidly increasing, and the price of oil peaked in April 1980 at over US$35 per barrel (equivalent to $115 per barrel in 2021 dollars term, when adjusted for inflation). Naturally, oil production increased and oil-producing countries found themselves fighting for market share. High prices and rising output were followed by a reduction in demand as industrial processes and automobiles were becoming more energy efficient. In addition, economic activity in industrial countries slowed due to the 1970s' financial crises, and in June 1981 *The New York Times* proclaimed that an "oil glut" had arrived. This oil glut was initially viewed as a temporary surplus, which later transformed into a 6-year decline in oil prices. From 1982 to 1985, the Organization for Petroleum Exporting Countries (OPEC) decreased oil production several times in order to stabilize prices, but these attempts failed as many OPEC members were producing above their quotas. Saudi Arabia was one of the few OPEC countries implementing output cuts, and soon non-OPEC countries surpassed OPEC in oil production levels. In 1986, Saudi Arabia grew tired of attempts to stabilize the market by curbing its output. In an about-face, they opened the spigot, increasing production from 2 million barrels per day to 5 million barrels per day. As a result, oil price fell during the first half of 1986 from US$27 to below US$10 ($67 to $25 in 2021 dollars term). The glut began in the early 1980s because of slowed economic activity in industrial countries due to the oil crises of the 1970s, especially in 1973 and 1979, and energy conservation spurred by high fuel prices [5].

The Gulf War is the third critical crisis which followed after the 1980s' oil glut, and this event had a significant influence on energy prices. In August of 1990, Iraq invaded Kuwait, reviving an old territorial dispute, and claimed that Kuwait was stealing its oil via slant drilling. As a result of this occupation, the price of Brent crude oil jumped from US$15 per barrel at the end of July 1990 to US$41.45 per barrel in October 1990. As oil production was slowing down in the Middle East due to tensions, and there was a potential risk to future oil supplies, the U.S. intervened and succeeded in removing Saddam Hussein's Iraqi forces from Kuwait,

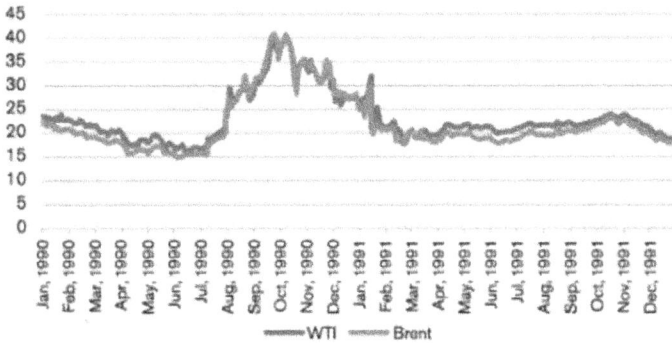

Figure 1. Crude spot prices during Gulf War.
Source: Major oil market crashes in history. Oil & Energy Online.

calming the oil market. The day after the U.S. and its allies launched an attack on Iraq, the oil price dropped 33% on 21 January 1991, which was the biggest daily decline at that time. The West Texas Intermediate (WTI) oil price retreated to the same level as it had been on 1 August 1990, one day before Iraq invaded Kuwait. Please refer to Figure 1 [6].

The 2008/09 Financial Crisis and the 2010 oil glut were the next significant events which had an enormous impact on energy prices. During the 2008/09 financial meltdown, the most significant long-term surge in oil prices transpired between 2003 and 2008 when WTI prices climbed from US$28 per barrel to US$134 per barrel. The jump in prices developed primarily from increases in demand in developing economies such as China and India. Weakness in the U.S. dollar and geopolitical tensions added fuel to the fire. In March 2008, OPEC accused the U.S. of economic "mismanagement" that was pushing prices to record highs. In June 2008, an Israeli attack on Iran caused yet another huge spike in the oil price. The highest price ever recorded for crude oil came in July 2008 when WTI crude reached a price of US$145.85 per barrel. Soon after, the 5-year price explosion ran its course when the global financial crises again drove down demand for crude oil just as additional supplies were ramping up. Prices plummeted from over US$100 per barrel to US$32. What

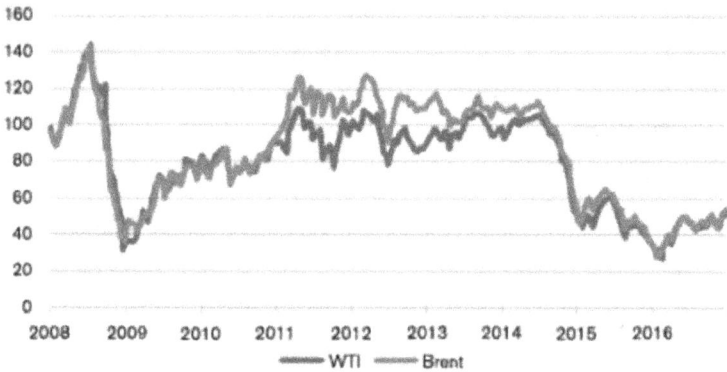

Figure 2. Crude oil spot prices 2008–2016.

Source: Major oil market crashes in history. Oil & Energy Online.

took 5 years to reach a crescendo was erased in less than 6 months. Like the 2008/09 Financial Crisis, the 2010 oil glut in keeping up with its penchant for financial market volatility and world crude prices made another march upward to over US$100 per barrel [7]. The difference here is that this time it took less than 2 years to get to that price level. However, higher prices inspired many to look for oil in hard-to-get places. In this sense, the shale revolution had begun. Fracking technology galvanized a black gold rush in unheard of places like Bakken, North Dakota. Meanwhile, the Canadians figured out how to get oil from sand in the backcountry of Alberta. The Saudi's once again made the regrettable decision to attempt to run the oil cowboys off the reservation by pumping more oil and driving prices low enough to drive them out of business. Ingenuity would prevail. Shale producers became more and more efficient. U.S. production quickly broke records. It took less than 2 years for the price to plunge from US$100 to US$26 per barrel. Please refer to Figure 2 [6].

3. Pandemic — Unprecedented Harbinger of Energy Crisis

As mentioned earlier, the Coronavirus Disease 2019, commonly known as the Covid-19 pandemic, is another cardinal event that is considered one of the most excruciating and has generated a traumatic economic impact and energy shocks in modern history. Severe impact on the global economy, including economies of the Association of South East Asian Nations (ASEAN), was inevitable. The economic slowdown arising from the pandemic appears to have affected the energy sector via two channels — the demand and supply sides. There has been a significant drop in energy demand during the Covid-19 pandemic. Due to concerns about public health and fearing that the increasing number of infected citizens would overwhelm national healthcare systems, countries introduced restrictions on both the international and internal movement of people to reduce the rate of spread of the disease. The rapid spread of the virus also led many countries to introduce lockdowns and other restrictive measures.

Being under lockdown generally had wide-ranging implications. Among other impacts, commercial activities were suspended apart from shopping at supermarkets and pharmacies, and working from home, where possible, became the standard. The lockdown measures in response to the global pandemic led to severe economic consequences. During the first year of the pandemic in 2020, worldwide demand for oil fell rapidly as governments across the globe closed businesses and restricted travel to contain the spread of the Covid-19 virus [8]. To illustrate this in more granular terms, the outbreak of Covid-19 and the wide-ranging measures needed to slow its advance triggered an unprecedented collapse in oil demand, a surge in oil inventories, and a record 1-month decline in oil prices on 21 April 2020, which saw WTI Crude Oil at US$11.26 a barrel. The oil industry was hit especially hard in 2020, forcing U.S. oil prices to go negative for the first time on record. Just a day before 21 April, in a matter of hours on 20 April 2020, the May 2020 contract futures price for WTI plummeted from US$18 a barrel to around negative US$37 a barrel. Oil producers were faced with a glut of crude oil that left them scrambling to find space to store the oversupply. Brent crude oil prices also tumbled, closing at US$9.12 a barrel on 21 April, a far cry from the US$70 a barrel that crude oil fetched at the beginning of the year. Although the plunge of U.S. oil futures into negative territory was short lived, the collapse in demand was extremely fast and volatile and the key lesson from this record plunge in oil prices was that it was predominantly driven by demand factors as wide-ranging measures to stem the pandemic precipitated an unprecedented collapse in oil demand, but the surge in oil inventories also exerted downward pressure on oil prices. Essentially, this sudden price drop in oil was the result of a direct confluence of macroeconomic factors in which the pandemic and the resulting economic shutdowns had drastically reduced the demand for oil, and the inventory tanks to store this oil supply were running out rapidly [9]. This insane occurrence of having a negative oil price was an outlier as insights into what exactly drove the market action that led to oil going into a negative territory discovered that there were a group of nine independent traders associated with Vega Capital London Limited who had the greatest impact on oil prices on 20 April 2020 [9].

While oil prices started strong in January 2020, by April, the impact of reduced economic activity created an oversupply and prices plunged dramatically. Adding to the free fall in oil prices was an oil price war between Saudi Arabia and Russia, initiated in March 2020 after the two countries failed to agree on oil production levels. The month-long price war ended in April when OPEC and its allies agreed to cut overall crude oil production by 9.7 million barrels per day for an initial period of 2 months, starting on 1 May 2020. This represented the single largest output cut in history. Oil production would be limited to 7.7 million barrels per day starting on 1 July and running through 31 December 2020. OPEC's failure to quickly cut oil production to respond to lower demand only added to the volatility and price declines that the oil industry experienced during the early part of the year (refer to Figure 3).

During the first 6 months of 2020, market uncertainties persisted for all energy sources, including liquid fuels, electricity, coal, natural gas, and renewables. Renewable energy projects experienced major delays and shutdowns as Covid-19 impacted major

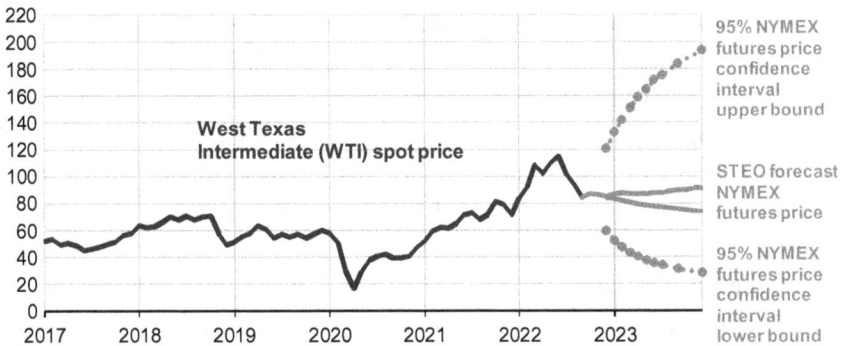

Figure 3. West Texas Intermediate (WTI) crude oil price and NYMEX confidence intervals.

Source: EIA [10].

industries, energy markets, and worker safety. Some of the halted renewable energy projects reported by the ASEAN Centre for Energy (ACE) in its "COVID-19 vs ASEAN Energy Sector: Renewables" report include the delay of the Philippines' 135-megawatt (MW) solar project, the shutting down of palm oil plants in Malaysia, and suspended hydropower construction by the Government of Laos, also known as Lao People's Democratic Republic [11]. The Covid-19 pandemic is indeed a crisis because it has placed the condition of the climate in uncertainty, slowing down energy transition, and disrupting the region's pursuit of energy security. But at the same time, it has provided an opportunity for ASEAN Member States (AMSs) to pave a different pathway to a greener and more sustainable energy future [12]. Covid-19 is an unprecedented crisis that has not only disrupted the supply chain of energy resources but has also forced nations to gravitate toward the development of their domestic energy sources.

Apart from the extensive disruptions to businesses and everyday life, there will also be longer-lasting consequences for the energy transition away from fossil fuels as fossil fuels are limited or not available for some countries, which has shifted the focus toward the development of renewable energy sources. This appears to have accelerated the energy transition to renewable energy that has already been under way. Put simply, in a post-pandemic era, this will lead governments to have an enormous reform capacity in terms of energy transition. Although the Covid-19 pandemic largely halted production and operations worldwide and resulted in widespread unemployment, it also provided chances to reshape the global economy and energy system. During the pandemic, governments have unprecedented implementation power to impose reform. The post-pandemic period is a precious opportunity for governments to enact legislations and regulations to compel energy-intensive companies to undertake structural adjustments so as to operate in an environment-friendly and low-carbon manner. According to an independent statistics and analytical study conducted by the U.S. Energy Information Administration [10], the EIA has forecast that the annual share of U.S. electricity generation from renewable energy sources will rise from 20% in 2021, to 22% in 2022, and to 23% in 2023, as a result of continuing increases in solar- and wind-generating capacities [10]. This increase in renewable generation leads to a decline in natural gas generation, which falls from a 37% share in 2021 to 35% in both 2022 and 2023 [10].

Furthermore, renewable energy has demonstrated several advantages during the pandemic, offering new insights for policymakers. On the one hand, air quality improved considerably during the Covid-19 lockdown, prompting people to be more conscious of environmental governance and clean energy [11]. Since renewable energy is clean and produces much less emissions than traditional energy, the renewable energy is recognized to be the key to improving air quality and public health. On the other hand, as most renewable energy sources can be remotely controlled and digitally intelligent, renewable energy plays a key role in maintaining a stable energy supply during Covid-19 [13]. For example, the combination of the Internet of Things (IoT) and renewable energy generation allows technicians to use cloud-based controllers to deploy distributed generation based on different stages of electricity demand [11,13]. Besides, based on sensors' perception of ambient environment information such as light intensity and wind speed, power generation equipment can also be started and stopped automatically, greatly improving energy efficiency and equipment life [11,13]. In contrast, traditional power generation is both energy- and labor-intensive, and the lack of fossil fuel supply and labor scarcity during the pandemic made it difficult to achieve an adequate supply of electricity. In addition, the use of renewable energy has also made significant contributions to pandemic control, for example, hydrogen-/solar-powered unmanned ground vehicles and their airborne counterparts can be used for search and rescue, and remote monitoring of urban ecosystems and agriculture production during lockdowns [13]. With tremendous reform capacity, governments can utilize these forward-thinking renewable energy technologies to open up a new path for energy transition.

While the pandemic has led to reductions in fossil fuel consumption and emissions, they will not be adequate to put the world on a path to meet the 2-degree global warming target, or drive coal consumption to near zero. To achieve the targets under the 2015 Paris Agreement as well as the more recent Conference of the Parties 26 (COP26) summit and limit global climate change, the energy transition will need to include a mosaic of solutions beyond just renewables and reducing fossil fuel consumption. Hydrogen, carbon capture utilization and storage (CCUS), biofuels, and even nuclear power are all likely to play significant roles in decarbonizing the interconnected global energy system. In this sense, the pandemic also appears to have pushed nations to focus on being more energy efficient through improving energy efficiency and demand-side management. For example, since the emergence of the Covid-19 outbreak, countries around the world were trying to cope and minimize the pandemic's impact on the industry sector. Physical distancing and working from home schemes have naturally affected many companies and the way they operate. To ease the pandemic impact, practicing energy efficiency and conservation (EE&C) measures were considered and adopted across the industry sectors [11]. During the 38th ASEAN Ministers Energy Meeting hosted virtually by Vietnam in November 2020, ASEAN has recognized the importance of emerging cross-sectoral imperatives, including economic recovery and digitalization [11]. The 6th ASEAN Energy Outlook analysis that was endorsed during the meeting also indicated about 70% potential final energy consumption savings from the transport and industry sectors, including potentially huge gains from further expanding the region's energy efficiency and conservation program [11]. Therefore, the strategy of economic recovery must also include investments in technological transformation in the industry sector, and several best practices to consider are Energy Management Systems and Virtual Desktop Infrastructure [11].

4. The Move Forward, Post-Covid-19 Energy Transition

The Covid-19 pandemic has created significant challenges for energy transition. Concerns about the overwhelming emphasis on economic recovery at the cost of energy transition progress have been raised worldwide. More voices are calling for "green" recovery initiatives, which recover the economy while not compromising our environment. This study thus provides a comprehensive analysis of the dynamics between energy transition and Covid-19 around the world and proposes a low-carbon energy transition roadmap in the post-pandemic era that has practical implications for green recovery initiatives in post-pandemic times.

4.1 *Energy Management System*

Energy Management System (EnMS) allows organizations to plan, organize, measure, control, and continuously improve the energy performance of its facilities, and this has been considered as a much-needed best practice since the emergence of the Covid-19 outbreak where both governments and companies globally have been trying to manage and reduce the pandemic's financial repercussions [11]. EnMS is a way of achieving energy efficiency through process optimization, and energy saving is one of the key efforts of every industry for its continual growth because of its great potential in cost reduction. Astra International, a multi-diversified Indonesian company, has opted for energy savings to survive the Covid-19 pandemic, compared to layoffs, as the company reported they could save up to US$8 million by implementing EnMS [11]. Astra also built their employees' awareness by the utilization of a smart timer to automate electricity usage. EnMS is a computer-based system that collects energy measurement data from devices and makes it available to users through online monitoring tools [11]. From the graphics or dashboards in the tool, users are able to monitor their energy consumption and improve energy efficiency. The use of EnMS in ASEAN is now growing rapidly in building smart cities to drive faster energy transition. For instance, an integrated district in Bangkok, Thailand, which includes office, housing, and hospital, was fully equipped with EnMS and centralized security [11].

Energy efficiency can also be applied in the production line. For instance, Pupuk Kaltim, an ammonia producer in Indonesia, has carried out factory energy management in its production efforts, through managing the quantity and proportion of ammonia produced and rescheduling turnaround time where it is appropriate to do so [11]. By saving energy, the company was able to lower operational costs and survive economically. This method is considered more effective with long-term benefits than lowering prices, reducing manufacturing outputs, or closing the factory completely.

While EnMS keeps tabs on energy expenditures and the energy savings potential, it is imperative that the use of technology in management and operations must also be environmentally friendly. To do this efficiently and effectively, organizations should also utilize building automation systems (BASs) as part of the whole suite of EnMS best practice to optimize heating, ventilation, air-conditioning, and lighting as well. BASs incorporate smart systems that draw on advanced technologies such as business intelligence and machine learning to evaluate the extent of energy utilized and improve efficiencies [11]. Some very good examples of BASs that have been utilized as part of the suite of EnMS to maximize energy efficiency can be seen in the case of the Kuala Lumpur International Airport in Malaysia as well as Changi Airport in Singapore [11].

4.2 *Virtual Desktop Infrastructure*

Another effective way of reducing energy consumption in offices and factories is by using Virtual Desktop Infrastructure (VDI). VDI is a standardized desktop environment using the organization's network that can be accessed by employees from anywhere. It not only provides simple desktop management and operation but also increases security, enhances flexibility, drives cost savings, simplifies information technology management as desktop environments are managed in one central location on a central server, and reduces the risk of systems' downtime. It comes with two options: Hybrid Cloud and Multi-cloud. Although these two terms are often used interchangeably, they possess a main difference in the location of non-cloud resources. Hybrid clouds utilize existing on-premises servers, storage, and networking, whereas in a multi-cloud (not hybrid) environment, those resources are also in the cloud, either at the same provider providing computing services or a co-location facility [11].

Research shows VDI can save up to 75% on hardware utilization, requires less power, and conserves nearly 90% energy footprint per user [11,12]. This technology could reduce costs while answering the accelerated demand from the organizations to comply with the work-from-home scheme, thus improving businesses' productivity. Building the infrastructure needed to support the digital world and subscribing to the latest technology have become very important for every business to stay competitive and run efficiently after Covid-19. Every organization must have a plan to anticipate unpredictable circumstances and events by ensuring availability, scalability, disaster recovery, and business continuity that does not depend on a single location. By implementing a Hybrid or Multi-cloud strategy, if there is a disruption in one cloud, resources can still be accessed by utilizing another cloud that is owned. The outbreak of the Covid-19 pandemic is an emergency that no country could anticipate. Nevertheless, industry sectors in Southeast Asia can overcome the crisis and come back stronger than before. Adapting and applying energy efficiency and conservation best practices in the management, operational, and building automation processes could accelerate business recovery.

These trends are expected to be permanent rather than transitory even after the Covid-19 pandemic ends and are posited as a new normal in the energy sector. A clean energy source holds an important role in the post-pandemic recovery. But the question lies in whether only renewables should be utilized or if another "clean" energy like nuclear could play a part in transitioning ASEAN's energy in a better way. This is especially important given the fact that several countries are interested in pursuing the nuclear option; for example, the Philippines is considering a revival of its dormant Bataan nuclear power plant [11,12].

4.3 *Variable renewable energy (VRE)*

Variable renewable energy (VRE) sources are just what the term sounds like: They produce renewable energy intermittently instead of on demand [14]. The large-scale deployment of solar and wind generation has altered the paradigm of power systems and electricity markets in which prices were traditionally based on marginal generation cost and fuel prices [14]. Most of the generation capacity was considered dispatchable and available throughout most of the year, and more importantly solar and wind do not require fuel and have practically zero marginal generation costs, as they are available only when the sun shines or when the wind blows [14].

Over the last two decades, VRE has experienced spectacular growth. In 2019 alone, the International Energy Agency (IEA) reported more than 100 gigawatts (GW) of completed solar photovoltaics (PV) and about 60 GW of completed wind power projects across the globe [12]. This was also highlighted by the remarkable journey of Vietnam with its 4.5-GW solar PV installation in 2019, surpassing Malaysia and Thailand in just 1 year. Also, both onshore and offshore wind projects are also gaining attention in Southeast Asia. Before the pandemic hit, in general VRE showed promising growth globally, including in the AMSs. However, there are technical challenges involved. Intermittency, grid stability, and technical and policy frameworks are the remaining obstacles that the AMSs need to resolve if the region wants to have a massive renewable energy injection [12]. Despite supply chain disruptions during the Covid-19 pandemic, the IEA recorded how VRE expansion increased renewable electricity generation by 5% in 2020. In an effort to accelerate decarbonization and energy transition, VRE development will continue to increase, especially in the Southeast Asian region [12].

4.4 *Nuclear energy*

On the contrary, nuclear energy has been underappreciated and has faced a lack of investment even before the Covid-19 pandemic. Despite being cheaper, more reliable, and having a smaller carbon footprint, countries often hesitate to develop nuclear energy due to its large initial investment and low public acceptance, according to ACE in its Civilian Nuclear Energy Factsheet. The 2011 Fukushima nuclear power accident in Japan raised even more concerns over the safety of nuclear power. Countries such as Germany, Belgium, Spain, and the United Kingdom aimed to phase out nuclear power completely by the mid-2020s to 2030s.

According to the IEA, only one new nuclear facility has been constructed over the past year, as opposed to 13 that have been permanently closed [15]. In Southeast Asia, the development of nuclear energy has been slow but steady, especially in Indonesia, Malaysia, Vietnam, Thailand, and the Philippines. As a result of the Covid-19 pandemic, nuclear power experienced a detrimental setback. Lower energy demand during the pandemic led to a reduction in nuclear power output, forcing the closure of nuclear reactors in Europe. Nevertheless, a lot of countries are still putting effort into pursuing nuclear project development, such as the United Arab Emirates (UAE), Pakistan, Turkey, Belarus, and some European countries. The World Nuclear Association (WNA) reported that about 100 reactors are under construction, increasing nuclear power capacity worldwide steadily [12]. Most planned reactors are in the Asian region, particularly in China, with some major plans for new units in Russia. In Southeast Asia, the Philippines is considering reviving a mothballed 621-megawatt electric (MWe) nuclear power plant. They have also issued a policy under Executive Order No. 116 as a major step toward the realization of the Philippines' nuclear energy program, indicating that nuclear energy is a promising option [12].

When Covid-19 forced countries into a lockdown for the first time, reports abounded of reduced pollution and clear skies as a result of the sharp reduction in economic activity, which has increased pressure on policymakers around the world to "build back better" by incorporating low-carbon, renewable energy sources like wind, solar, and hydropower into the energy mix. As a small, resource-constrained city-state, however, Singapore imports almost all of its energy needs and has limited renewable energy options [16–18]. Imported natural gas generates 95% of Singapore's electricity, and 80% of the total electricity produced is used to power Singapore's industrial and commercial sectors, with household and transport-related uses accounting for the remainder. Here, the country's overreliance on imported natural gas for electricity leaves it vulnerable to price shocks and supply disruptions [16–18]. The ongoing pandemic has laid bare the volatility of oil markets and confirmed that electricity supplies are crucial to all aspects of life in a wired economy, including the need to be able to work from home. In order to mitigate the effects of future shocks, Singapore would be well advised to consider incorporating alternative energy sources suitable for Singapore's needs, and nuclear energy warrants a closer look [16–19].

The idea of using nuclear energy for the island state is not new. Back in 2008, Singapore's late Minister Mentor Lee Kuan Yew communicated that he once contemplated nuclear energy to be the best alternative to fossil fuels for Singapore, and it is not difficult to comprehend why [20]. Located in the tropics, the island-state has a high dependence on air-conditioning and the variability in Singapore's electricity demand is much lower as compared to other countries, which makes the case for a low-carbon baseload electricity supply typical of nuclear energy generation [20]. Bringing nuclear energy into Singapore would also boost the country's energy and engineering sectors while potentially creating thousands of high-skilled jobs [16,17,19,20]. Today, nuclear provides 10% of the world's electricity, but expansion has been slow as the technology faces many formidable obstacles [20]. Nuclear power plants are costly to build, prone to construction delays and cost overruns, and endure exorbitant regulatory costs in addition to negative public perception [18,21]. Indeed, fear of radiation is widespread, yet the truth is that much of this fear is unfounded. Taking a transcontinental flight or getting medical scans can expose a person to more radiation than living within a 50-mile radius of a nuclear power plant [20,21]. Despite sharply polarized opinions toward nuclear energy post Fukushima, the AMSs remain interested in it, given its strategic relevance in the region's energy and climate targets as concluded in a study by the Energy Studies Institute (ESI) at the National University of Singapore (NUS) in 2014 [12,20]. After all, nuclear power is one of the cleanest forms of energy besides wind and solar and it is a reliable energy alternative and more importantly is considered as a low-carbon energy source [12,16,17,19,20].

Arguably, the upcoming hydrogen revolution and carbon capture technologies are among the more publicly acceptable approaches to decarbonization for the moment. But Singapore faces unique adoption challenges, including a lack of land space. Considering the urgency of global climate challenge, it would be unwise to exclude available technologies like nuclear power from decarbonization efforts. The introduction of small modular reactors (SMRs) then promises to reinvent nuclear power for the modern era. These are miniaturized nuclear power plants, operating on the same principle as large ones, have several key advantages [16,17,19]. Consider a small yacht and a large cruise ship: The yacht would be a lot easier to build, given its mass and size, control, and maintain as compared to the cruise ship, albeit catering to a homogenous consumer group but with marginally different expectations [20].

4.5 *ASEAN's green recovery path and nuclear energy*

Global opinion on nuclear energy has always been misplaced due to focused attention on its production and the use of radioactive fuels. However, nuclear power has the highest capacity factor (CF), thus creating a low-carbon source of baseload energy. There are several reasons why nuclear should be included in the green recovery path post the pandemic.

First, switching coal to nuclear for baseload is far more efficient as it decarbonizes as much as wind power does. Nuclear power plants only release greenhouse gas (GHG) emissions during ancillary use of fossil fuels, such as during construction, mining, fuel processing, maintenance, and decommissioning. Second, nuclear power plants operate at a much higher CF compared to other renewables, let alone fossil fuels. The U.S. Energy Information Administration (EIA) recorded the CF of nuclear power at 93.5% in 2019, much higher than all other energy sources [10]. This means nuclear power is a definite winner in terms of baseload reliability, which is a great replacement for coal in continuous operation to meet minimum electricity demands. Third, countries such as Indonesia, Malaysia, Vietnam, Thailand, and the Philippines already have good knowledge of and capacity for nuclear power due to their years of research. Besides, the 6th ASEAN Energy Outlook projected a huge increase in ASEAN's residential electricity demand, reaching 497.1 terawatt hour (TWh) by 2040 [12].

The basis of using nuclear energy is this: Instead of building coal power plants where obtaining financing is becoming increasingly difficult, nuclear can be a viable option to providing clean electricity on a large scale [12]. Nuclear power plants use less land to generate electricity compared to other clean energy sources, as stated by ACE in the Civilian Nuclear Energy Factsheet [12,19]. It is a reliable source of energy as well as being a cost-effective solution in the right manner. Furthermore, the development of nuclear energy can boost ASEAN's job opportunities and support regional energy security [19]. It is commendable that many countries are trying to prioritize VRE in their respective recovery paths. However, because we need massive amounts of electricity to meet the demands of post-Covid-19 global economic recovery in a short period, nuclear should be on the table in tandem with VRE, replacing fossil fuels as the source of baseload energy [12]. To pursue the nuclear option, governments need to prepare frameworks to enable suitable environments, as well as enhancing nuclear technology capacity. Also, the AMSs need to learn from other countries' experiences, benchmarking with other successful nuclear pioneers, especially in changing public perception toward nuclear.

Recently, there has been a strong interest in small and medium-sized modular reactors, driven by the desire to reduce capital cost and to provide power in remote areas. Small modular reactors (SMRs) can accommodate flexible power generation for a wider range of applications with a capacity of 300 MWe per unit [12]. Also, they display an enhanced safety performance and offer the possibility for synergetic hybrid energy systems, including the combination of nuclear and VRE [12,18]. Nuclear power, together with VRE, can help the AMSs ensure grid reliability without compromising affordability [12]. Thus, energy transition in the region could run smoothly and help it to build back better in the post-pandemic era.

5. Conclusion

The present pandemic has given us glimpses of what the future of the energy sector will bring, and the glimpses keep changing as the Covid-19 crisis continues with no early end in sight. A host of cost pressures brought about by the surge in economic activity, rising commodity prices, and global supply chain disruptions during the Covid-19 pandemic have been passed on to consumers around the globe in the form of higher prices of goods and services across the board [22]. The latest wave of Covid-19 infections in Mainland China and the continuous pursuance of a zero Covid-19 strategy coupled with extreme controls and lockdowns have dealt a heavy blow to China's economy and have also threatened to worsen the disruption in the global supply chain [22,23]. While there were preliminary hopes that this global inflationary pressure would ease, economists now expect these global inflationary pressures to persist over the long term due to the Russia–Ukraine war that has been ongoing since 24 February 2022 [22].

There are two general themes that run through this chapter, reflecting that we are still in the middle of a global crisis. One is that uncertainty about the longer term is even greater than usual because we do not know how governments and consumers are going to behave in a post-Covid-19 world. The other is the tension between short-term imperatives (financial stresses) and the longer-term need for investment and adaptation that is also unusually high. While some believe that stimulus measures to limit the human and economic impact of the Covid-19 pandemic offer a chance to rebuild a cleaner and more sustainable world, others are more skeptical. There also seems to be an acceptance that the pace of the clean energy transition in a post-Covid-19 world will not be uniform across the globe and that weakened international cooperation reduces the chance of fast-tracking the low-carbon transition globally. While the world has made important strides toward clean energy transition in the past decade, there is still a long way to go. As global energy transition advances together with the ongoing global recovery efforts from the Covid-19 pandemic, there are some key takeaways as to how the new normal will pan out for the energy sector in a post-Covid-19 world.

First, energy remains strongly linked with economic growth [24]. Despite the historic emissions reductions caused by lockdowns, emissions in many countries rebounded to pre-pandemic levels quickly [25]. Moreover, as a huge financial outlay is being pledged and effectively allocated to sectors relevant to energy transition, a majority of those resources have been allocated to carbon-intensive sectors in most countries, potentially locking in emissions for years. Investment in green, future-ready infrastructure can be a strong vehicle to drive further economic growth and generate employment.

Second, not all economic recoveries will support this energy transition equally in a post-Covid-19 world [26]. As the global economy works toward normalcy, forecasts suggest that developing economies are on track for slower recovery, with many not expected to return to pre-pandemic GDP levels until 2023, according to the International Monetary Fund (IMF) [26]. The prospect of divergent economic recovery, and resulting fiscal challenges, will limit their ability to support investments into energy transition. In the short term, ramping up vaccine production and distribution, and ensuring equitable distribution, is important to ensure emerging and developing economies are quickly able to bounce back.

Finally, challenges in international collaboration remain. The Covid-19 pandemic revealed the limitations of international cooperation to mitigate the global health emergency quickly. Climate change, the primary driver of energy transition, has already created food and water shortages across many parts of the world and is expected to spark an unprecedented wave of bigger problems in the near future, if left unaddressed. Given the ubiquitous presence of energy across the facade of every modern economy and society, clean energy transition has systemic implications and requires active participation from all in a post-Covid-19 world.

References

[1] IEA. (2022). International Energy Agency. Retrieved from: https://www.iea.org/. Accessed on 28 April 2022.

[2] Martin, E., Fergal, O. B., and Nardelli, A. (2020). IMF warns against premature withdrawal of stimulus amid Covid resurgence. Bloomberg. Retrieved from: https://www.business-standard.com/article/international/imf-warns-against-premature-withdrawal-of-stimulus-amid-covid-resurgence-120112000030_1.html. Accessed on 29 April 2022.

[3] Roose, K. D. (1954). *The Economics of Recession and Revival: An Interpretation of 1937–38*. New Haven: Yale University Press.

[4] Masterson, V. (2022). The 1973 energy crisis sparked the idea for establishing the IEA. What have we learned since? World Economic Forum. Retrieved from: https://www.weforum.org/agenda/2022/03/iea-1970s-energy-crisis/. Accessed on 27 April 2022.

[5] Richards, H. (2022). What the 1970s teaches about today's energy crisis. Energy Wire News. Retrieved from: https://www.eenews.net/articles/what-the-1970s-teaches-about-todays-energy-crisis/. Accessed on 27 April 2022.

[6] Ristanovic, A. (2022). Major oil market crashes in history. Oil & Energy Online. Retrieved from: https://oilandenergyonline.com/articles/all/major-oil-market-crashes-history/. Accessed on 27 April 2022.

[7] Hershey, Jr. and Robert, D. (1981). How the oil glut is changing business. The New York Times. Accessed on 27 April 2022.

[8] Eberhart, D. (2021). Energy crisis threatens return of 1970s inflation. Forbes Energy. Retrieved from: https://www.forbes.com/sites/daneberhart/2021/10/19/energy-crisis-threatens-return-of-1970s-inflation/?sh=545d37f77e20. Accessed on 27 April 2022.

[9] Vaughan, L., Chellel, K., and Bain, B. (2020). The Essex Boys: How nine traders hit a gusher with negative oil. Bloomberg Businessweek Feature. Retrieved from: https://www.bloomberg.com/news/features/2020-12-10/stock-market-when-oil-when-negative-these-essex-traders-pounced. Accessed on 29 April 2022.

[10] EIA. (2022). U.S. Energy Information Administration. Independent Statistics & Analysis. Retrieved from: https://www.eia.gov/outlooks/steo/. Accessed on 27 April 2022.

[11] Fatika, H. L. and Safrina, R. (2021). Energy efficiency as the industry's way to survive the Covid-19 crisis. ASEAN Climate Change and Energy Project. Retrieved from: https://accept.aseanenergy.org/energy-efficiency-as-the-industrys-way-to-survive-the-covid-19-crisis/. Accessed on 28 April 2022.

[12] Shani, N. (2021). Nuclear energy in a post-pandemic ASEAN. The ASEAN Post. Retrieved from: https://theaseanpost.com/article/nuclear-energy-post-pandemic-asean. Accessed on 28 April 2022.

[13] Tian, J. F., Yu, L. G., Xue, R., Zhuang, S., and Shan, Y. L. (2022). Global low-carbon energy transition in the post-Covid-19 era. *Applied Energy*, **307**(118205). https://doi.org/10.1016/j.apenergy.2021.118205. Accessed on 13 May 2022.

[14] IRENA. (2022). International Renewable Energy Agency: Variable renewable energy. Retrieved from: https://www.irena.org/power/Variable-Renewable-Energy. Accessed on 29 April 2022.

[15] Varro, L. and Fraser, P. (2020). The Covid-19 crisis is undermining nuclear power's important role in clean energy transitions. International Energy Agency (IEA). Retrieved from: https://www.iea.org/commentaries/the-covid-19-crisis-is-undermining-nuclear-power-s-important-role-in-clean-energy-transitions. Accessed on 29 April 2022.

[16] Ang, Q. (2022). Singapore explores tapping nuclear energy by 2050. The Straits Times. Retrieved from: https://www.straitstimes.com/singapore/environment/singapore-exploring-tapping-nuclear-energy-by-2050. Accessed on 27 April 2022.

[17] Cheah, M. (2022). Singapore still considering deployment of nuclear, geothermal energy: Alvin Tan. The Business Times. Retrieved from: https://www.businesstimes.com.sg/government-economy/singapore-still-considering-deployment-of-nuclear-geothermal-energy-alvin-tan. Accessed on 28 April 2022.

[18] Yeoh, G. (2022). New technologies have potential to make futures nuclear power plants "much safer" than existing ones: MTI. Channel NewsAsia. Retrieved from: https://www.channelnewsasia.com/singapore/new-nuclear-energy-technologies-potential-much-safer-mti-2606196. Accessed on 28 April 2022.

[19] Muruganathan, K. (2022). What it means to have nuclear energy in Singapore power sector's net zero emission aim. Today. Retrieved from: https://www.todayonline.com/commentary/what-it-means-have-nuclear-energy-singapore-power-sectors-net-zero-emission-aim-1860286. Accessed on 28 April 2022.

[20] Nian, V. and Goh, G. (2020). Why Singapore should consider nuclear power. Sustainability Times. Retrieved from: https://www.sustainability-times.com/clean-cities/why-singapore-should-consider-nuclear-power/. Accessed on 27 April 2022.

[21] Chandler, D. L. (2020). Study identifies reasons for soaring nuclear plant cost overruns in the U.S. MIT News. Retrieved from: https://news.mit.edu/2020/reasons-nuclear-overruns-1118. Accessed on 28 April 2022.

[22] Awang, N. (2022). The big read: With inflation putting the squeeze on families, some give up the frills while others cut back on basics. Channel NewsAsia. Retrieved from: https://www.channelnewsasia.com/singapore/big-read-inflation-cost-living-families-money-finances-income-rising-prices-2617781. Accessed on 29 April 2022.

[23] Bradsher, K. (2022). China's Covid lockdowns set to further disrupt global supply chains. Retrieved from: https://www.nytimes.com/2022/03/15/business/covid-china-economy.html. Accessed on 28 April 2022.

[24] Sharma, N., Smeets, B., and Tryggestad, C. (2019). The decoupling of GDP and energy growth: A CEO guide. McKinsey Quarterly: McKinsey & Company. Retrieved from: https://www.mckinsey.com/industries/electric-power-and-natural-gas/our-insights/the-decoupling-of-gdp-and-energy-growth-a-ceo-guide. Accessed on 29 April 2022.

[25] Januta, A. (2021). Global carbon emissions rebound to near pre-pandemic levels. Reuters. Retrieved from: https://www.reuters.com/

business/cop/global-carbon-emissions-rebound-near-pre-pandemic-levels-2021-11-04/. Accessed on 29 April 2022.

[26] Singh, H. V. and Gomez, P. (2021). 5 key lessons for energy transition from Covid-19 recovery. World Economic Forum. Retrieved from: https://www.weforum.org/agenda/2021/04/5-key-lessons-for-energy-transition-from-covid-19-recovery/. Accessed on 29 April 2022.

Chapter 4

Transformation and Reshaping of Industrial Supply Chains in the Post-Pandemic Era

Zhang Meilin

Singapore University of Social Sciences, Singapore

1. Introduction

In the past 3 years, the pandemic has had a significant impact on global supply chains. The outbreak and recurring cycles have triggered problems, causing intermittent shutdowns in many industries, further exacerbating supply chain challenges caused by world trade conflicts and rising global manufacturing costs [1]. Under the influence of the epidemic, the supply chain of the global industrial manufacturing industry has been severely impacted. According to our research and observations in several industries, the supply chain of manufacturing enterprises is facing more challenges: shrinking global market demand and declining mid-end revenue, the production of factories having been suspended or reduced due to limited resumption of work, the supply of raw materials or parts being in shortage, labor shortages, logistics disruptions or reduced efficiency, out-of-stocks or backlogs of finished goods due to unexpected order changes, and defaults due to inability to meet contracts on time [2]. The supply chain challenges of industrial enterprises are rapidly spreading to the entire industrial value chain and the global supply chain.

The post-epidemic era has far-reaching impacts on the global value chain system, and the specific impacts are mainly reflected at the enterprise and country levels:

- At the corporate level, the Covid-19 pandemic has brought huge losses to companies in the global industrial value chain, forcing companies to pay special attention to supply chain risks and rethink their supply chain layout [3].

As the pandemic has caused economic shutdowns around the world, a large number of companies that rely on the global "Just-In-Time" operation are facing "manufacturing deserts", supply chain failures, and disconnection between production and sales [4]. According to the McKinsey report, the total value of global merchandise trade affected by this has reached the level of US$2.9 trillion to US$4.6 trillion, which is equivalent to the total global merchandise trade compared with 2018 data. It can be seen that the enterprises whose production layout is based on the global value chain have been greatly impacted in this process [5].

Huge losses force companies to rethink how to avoid related risks in the future, which abruptly increases the importance of supply chain security in its strategic development planning, and companies will reconsider the layout of the supply chain accordingly in the future. Thus, the pandemic has had a significant impact on the risk appetite of these enterprises. One of the most noteworthy findings is that the importance of supply chain security has risen from the ninth place before the outbreak to the second after the outbreak. Now, it is one of the risks that most concerns the executives of enterprises. And many more companies will focus on reconfiguring their supply chains in the future:

- At the national level, while the Covid-19 epidemic has brought great damage to the economies of various countries, it has also made governments realize the importance of a complete industrial chain system.

After the outbreak, due to the different stages of development of the pandemic, the time intervals for entering the economic shutdown were also different. For the global supply chain, the industrial links distributed in various countries in the world were located in specific positions in the industrial chain, including both the production link and the consumption link. Each link was shut down in batches, making the industrial chain unable to operate in a complete form. Therefore, the actual operation efficiency of these industries has never reached the normal level, and even if some countries have certain production links in a specific industrial chain, they still cannot complete the normal production process when other countries are shut down and the chain is broken, which has caused the governments of various countries to pay special attention to the construction of the integrity, security, and sustainability of the industrial chain, and this is precisely the impact of the pandemic on the national strategy or policy level of the global industrial chain system [6].

From the mid-21st century, the industrial division of labor and trade based on the global value chain has undergone profound changes, and the regionalization trend of the value chain pattern has become more obvious. A prominent change is that China's position in the global value chain division of labor has significantly improved. At present, the global supply chain has gradually formed a "three centers" pattern with the United States, Germany, and China as the local cores. Among them, the United States and Germany are mainly characterized by high-tech industries and innovation, while China is characterized by manufacturing and consumer markets, and is gradually shifting toward high-tech. In this process, China and the United States will maintain a certain supply chain connection for a long time, but the competition between the two sides in the high-tech field will be more intense. Under the impact of external factors such as Sino–US trade friction and the new regional crisis, countries have increasingly paid attention to the risk that the industrial chain of key industries is too concentrated overseas or in a certain region and raised supply chain security and risk to the highest strategic level.

To this end, supply chain leaders have focused on the post-pandemic era and begun to decentralize manufacturing, increase automation, and create a more customer-centric supply chain.

Improving the resilience and flexibility of supply chains not only helps organizations cope with environmental changes but also enables organizations to turn crisis into opportunity and achieve long-term competitive advantage. In the current environment, supply chain leaders must view the supply chain from a systems perspective [7].

2. The Trends and Determinants of the Global Industrial Chain before the Pandemic

After World War II, with emerging market countries participating in internationalization in all aspects, foreign direct investment from developed countries had grown substantially, and more companies began to use global supply chains to organize production. Therefore, in order to decipher the key factors, it is necessary to find the development trend and determinants of the global industrial chain before the epidemic.

- The primary reason is that under the premise of global economic development, enterprises pursue low cost and high efficiency. They carry out labor-intensive production in low-cost areas such as labor and warehousing, and split production links to achieve profitability in the global value chain by controlling transportation costs. The company's comparative advantage in cost efficiency becomes the most critical factor in the expansion phase. Multinational enterprises, which are practitioners of global cost-effectiveness strategy, have become the core carriers for the realization of the global industrial chain layout, vigorously driving the rapid growth of the scale of the global value chain and building the traditional supply chain on a globalized structure.
- Another reason is the continuous development of science and technology, especially the level of information technology which makes it possible to closely coordinate information and logistics in different countries and time zones and objectively provides the necessary conditions for the formation of global value

chains. Driven by "profit maximization," most corporate factories adopt the principle of Just-in-Time Manufacturing, reducing inventory to optimize the cost derived from idle resources. Not only that, one of the purposes of globalization is to use the comparative advantages of each country to produce or provide goods and services in a certain link in the supply chain, and then obtain maximum efficiency and profit through international trade, creating the current supply chain. The chain is a highly globalized and transnational division of labor [5].

- The third reason is that global trade barriers are still at a relatively low stage, and public health epidemics occasionally occur, but they have never become as serious as the global epidemic of new coronavirus in 2020! The trade protectionism policies of various countries have not yet prevailed, and the manufacturing and logistics of raw materials, intermediate products, and finished products around the world are relatively smooth. Therefore, enterprises in various countries do not need to consider the risks and restrictions brought about by geopolitics. Low cost and high efficiency are the most important development principles, providing the necessary conditions for the development of global value chains [8].

With the increasing escalation of the Sino–US trade war, the expansion phase of the global value chain has basically ended, and it has entered a stage of maturity or even decline. The vast majority of this adjustment process is still cost driven. After decades of development, industries that are relatively suitable for production decentralization under the premise of comparative cost advantages have basically completed this transformation, and there are fewer and fewer industries that still need new supply chain layouts globally. Therefore, the global expansion of value chain will be limited.

On the other hand, with the development of automated production technology, the labor cost advantage of developing countries is no longer obvious. With the advancement of science and technology in the field of mechanization and automated production, the cost saved by enterprises through the application of the global supply chain, that is, the difference between the wages and transportation costs of low-wage countries relative to the domestic market of enterprises, is newly achieved by using more robots to replace production workers. All these make enterprises lose the motivation to disperse production links in developing countries with lower costs.

When more extreme uncertain challenges arrive, based on the existing development trend of the global industrial chain before the epidemic, combined with the impact of the pandemic on the industrial system, it can be predicted that the future development direction of the global industrial chain will change from the previous cost efficiency. The security factor dominates and it will be transformed into a dual drive that takes into account stability and efficiency, and the risk management model will also undergo great changes. Industrial companies need to focus on development and innovation in four areas: supply diversity, value chain competitiveness, and green and low-carbon productions.

3. Supply Chain Diversity/Resilience

Many companies intentionally design appropriate redundancy into their supply chain operations. The epidemic crisis revealed that the main reason for the suspension of production due to the interruption of the supply chain of industrial enterprises during the epidemic is that the supply source is too concentrated. The epidemic has taught a lesson to many multinational companies that focusing only on efficiency and cost is far from enough, as "flexibility" or supply chain robustness under uncertainty is critical, which may not guarantee cost efficiency. Therefore, companies have to make trade-offs and sacrifice some efficiency in return for the resilience. Because, when there is disruption upstream of the supply chain, it will definitely affect the downstream. For example, the shortage of raw materials will interrupt production, and a delay in the delivery of finished products will cause the market to be out of stock, which will eventually affect other nodes in the supply chain such as sales. This "linear" characteristic makes supply chains structurally inflexible to respond to increasing contingencies. In addition, the design of the traditional supply chain structure also has the various defects, so that the resilience of the current supply chain is limited, and any sudden interruption will threaten the end-to-end stability of the overall supply chain.

The pandemic will prompt countries and companies to accelerate their shift to regional supply chains and reverse the process of globalization. Among them, the supply chain network in Asia, the global manufacturing hub, will become more diverse. In addition to this, companies should also reduce their reliance on any single supplier if they want to reduce the risk of supply chain disruption, but diversification also does not protect companies from systemic risks such as a pandemic.

Through an extensive number of case studies, we found that companies can consider the following two main ways to improve the diversity of their supply chains.

3.1 *Establish a regionalized supply chain base to reduce dependence on a single region*

For example, a global chemical company has always relied on the United States as a global supply base for its upstream product integration. In order to increase the diversity of its supply chain, this industry-leading company has established multiple regional supply chain bases in the United States, the Middle East, and the Asia-Pacific region. In order to balance the layout of the regional supply chain and reduce the overreliance on the US supply chain base, the company implemented a regional supply chain center that is "based in Asia, serving Asia," and redesigned its regional production capacity and network, including the Asia-Pacific region, of factories and distribution networks [5].

Another example we cite here is a global clothing brand. The company purchases raw materials from hundreds of suppliers in 11 countries, and more than half of the suppliers are located in China, Vietnam, and India. The network effectively enhances its cross-regional supply risk capability.

Decentralized manufacturing and supplier diversification have become priorities for many executives, both in response to the trade war and in the desire to create a more agile supply chain. Decentralized manufacturing is a top priority for its customers today too. "The need for decentralized manufacturing is more pressing, it's happening, and it's happening faster." Finally, companies need to strengthen the resilience of their organizations and partner networks, especially the financial health of companies within their supply chain ecosystems.

3.2 Strengthen the self-organization of the supply chain

The ability of a supply chain system to correct itself largely depends on its ability to self-organize and resume normal operations when a feedback loop is received. If companies can quickly sense and anticipate the challenges posed by the Covid-19 pandemic, they are bound to go further.

Businesses that lack such feedback loops struggle to respond quickly to changing customer needs. An executive of a global consumer goods technology company pointed out that companies with overly concentrated decision-making power cannot effectively respond to the new epidemic crisis.

According to a KPMG report [8],

> "It is difficult for us to respond quickly, all decision-making power is concentrated in headquarters, and the problem is that they often do not understand the specific situation of the locality. Many times, we need to explain the background, the problem, the options and the offer bit by bit. Communication takes a lot of time and prevents us from moving quickly."

Dave Ingram, Chief Procurement Officer at Unilever, has a similar opinion: "The centralized model makes the decision-making process too long, so we must put more power delegated to the team in charge."

Decentralization helps improve the efficiency of feedback loops and builds the ability for teams to self-organize, while centralization can be counterproductive. A self-organizing system can withstand a certain amount of chaos and error. "In Flextronics, making mistakes is not a problem, because our corporate culture provides those who are recognized with the opportunity to try and make mistakes." Chen Guanghui (Flextronics) also pointed out, "Everyone can come up with a better plan, but if there is no corresponding corporate culture support, then plans can only stay on paper forever" [9].

With the spread of the epidemic in the early stage, companies increasingly need to respond flexibly to unconventional situations according to local policies. The increase in market emergencies will undoubtedly increase the uncertainty of supply and demand in the future industry supply chain. A series of supply chain management challenges caused by the epidemic include suspension or shortage of upstream supply, increased safety requirements, and inability to resume production at full capacity, which worsen the operation as labor shortages lead to increased labor costs, logistics disruptions lead to increased costs and longer cycle times, etc.

In the face of challenges, enterprises need to improve the ability of the supply chain to efficiently respond to changes on the basis of increasing procurement flexibility, manufacturing flexibility, and logistics flexibility.

4. Competitiveness of the Value Chain

Improving the competitiveness of the value chain is mainly through the integration of the value chain, divesting or outsourcing non-core operations. Taking Chinese manufacturing enterprises as an example, most small and medium-sized enterprises generally dominate low-end value production links, but the core technical capabilities of high value-added upstream R&D design, or key upstream raw materials and core components, are often controlled by others. The downstream brand and channel links also rarely have strong control ability and the ability to obtain higher brand and channel premium. Many enterprises are big but not strong, and have not yet broken through the shackles of weak positioning in the industrial value chain. On the other hand, traditional manufacturing enterprises have also failed to identify and strengthen their core competitiveness, and often invest limited resources in non-core businesses or operational links, stretching the front line too long. The epidemic has impacted the normal operation of many industrial enterprises, but it has also made enterprises more aware of their own shortcomings and real gaps in core competitiveness.

At the same time, the digital supply chain meets the requirements of the new form of supply chain development. Digital transformation enables individuality, customization, flexibility, agility, and resilience. The digital supply chain is the application of cutting-edge technologies such as artificial intelligence, big data, cloud computing, and blockchain, as well as the transformation and upgrading of the traditional production model. In addition, the new epidemic has created a large number of non-contact digital application scenarios. At the same time, the fragmentation of the global market has also put forward higher requirements for the level of digitalization of the supply chain. Only through digital transformation can we cope with uncertainty and make mass customized production possible.

Additionally, more and more companies are investing in digital and data analytics capabilities to help local teams gain business intelligence and consumer insights. Ingram said that its company has already started to use "insight engine," which aims to understand consumption motivation through data and ultimately shape corporate strategy. Large multinational corporations such as General Mills are also beginning to take a longer-term view of supply chain technology in response to the next crisis. Fu Jianjun, Head of Integrated Supply Chain at General Mills China, pointed out, "We are building direct-to-consumer (DTC) capabilities while improving data and analytics capabilities." Huang Hong added, "Data is king! Data authenticity, data analysis capability and usability are critical for business." [8]

From many more industry practices today, digitization, especially through the direct penetration of the entire supply chain information, helps the domestic supply chain structure develop in the direction of the entire industry chain (upstream and downstream enterprises). This strategy increases a company's competitive advantages in the long run.

5. Green and Low-Carbon Supply Chain

Issues such as global climate change, environmental pollution, and resource scarcity are common challenges faced by mankind. The green development of the supply chain is of great significance for promoting the green development of the global economy. Since 2018, nearly 130 countries and regions have committed to carbon neutrality through legislation and policy announcements [7].

Building a green supply chain is not only an important part of a green, low-carbon, and circular development of an economic system but also a reflection of the core competitiveness of future enterprises. The U.S. Clean Energy Revolution and Environmental Justice Initiative requires public companies to disclose climate risks and greenhouse gas emissions in their operations and supply chains. The European Commission passed the EU Climate Law, which enshrines the European Union's political commitment to remain climate neutral by 2050. Major companies in various countries have put forward carbon peaking and carbon neutrality target times, and pay attention to carbon emissions in the supply chain. For companies that do not meet green and low carbon standards, they will face high carbon tariffs.

For both enterprises and a majority of developing countries, green supply chain is the only way to develop a sustainable global economy in the post-pandemic era.

Enterprises should make full use of the national policy opportunity to adjust and optimize the industrial structure and energy structure, actively eliminate outdated production capacity, realize the green and intelligent development of the supply chain, and finally form the modern layout and strategic goal of the enterprise supply chain. Enterprises should also improve the flexibility of the green supply chain of enterprises by participating in the trading of carbon emission rights and pollution rights. Using environmental labeling of products, green product certification systems, and subscribing for enterprise "green certificates" may help enterprises to expand the green consumer market and strengthen the competitiveness of enterprises' green supply chain. In the enterprise culture reshaping, one should integrate the concept of green development into the economic development after the epidemic, and increase the inclination toward green projects in the new investment.

As for how to build a green governance mechanism, we recommend that one focus on two aspects. First, all involved companies should set up internal green management systems of the enterprise, including green management positions, green management systems, and green compliance mechanisms, connecting with the national ecological industry innovation evaluation system, ecological certification system, ecological statistics system, ecological audit system, ecological verification system, property rights protection system, and other systems. Second, they need to have an ecological value realization mechanism. This is the dynamic mechanism for the transformation of ecological resources into ecological assets and ecological capital.

6. Conclusion

The post-pandemic era has arrived, and geopolitical conflicts and economic frictions have forced companies to reassess and restructure their supply chains. Leaders need to build resilience in their supply chains and improve the competitiveness of their products and services in order to effectively respond to uncertain emergencies and crises. At the same time, one should always put customers at the core of supply strategy, embrace technology and designate corresponding crisis plans, so as to have the ability and influence to build a strong supply chain and calmly deal with current challenges and future crises [9].

If enterprises can strategize, plan ahead, and make relevant preparations, they will not only be able to effectively and quickly undertake new opportunities for creative services under the trend of new industrial chains in the post-epidemic era but also contribute to the development of an innovative industrial network system.

As carbon regulations and market risks become more and more significant, companies must integrate greenery in their business strategy, technology research, and development as well as the overall industrial chain. In order to assess the effectiveness and enthusiasm of enterprises in managing their own environmental impacts, we analyzed which enterprises are more likely to compete for low-carbon transformation in the future from a series of indicators such as corporate governance, strategy, risk management, carbon emission measurement, and energy conservation and emission reduction actions. We found that regulatory and financial risk impacts far outweigh opportunities, and there are still significant gaps in opportunity identification and practice.

References

[1]   Cordon, C. and Buatois, E. (2020). A post COVID-19 outlook: The future of the supply chain. IMD — International Institute for Management Development. https://www.imd.org/research-knowledge/articles/A-post-COVID-19-outlook-The-future-of-the-supply-chain/.

[2]   Jensen, H. H. (2020). How global trade digitization could support COVID-19's economic rebound. World Economic Forum, April 2020. https://www.weforum.org/agenda/2020/04/global-trade-digitization-covid-19-economic-rebound-blockchain-toolkit.

[3]   Lin, J. and Lanng, C. (2020). Here's how global supply chains will change after COVID-19. World Economic Forum, May 2020. https://www.weforum.org/agenda/2020/05/this-is-what-global-supply-chains-will-look-like-after-covid-19/.

[4]   Kilic, K. and Marin, D. (2020). How COVID-19 is transforming the world economy. VoxEU.org, 10 May 2020.

[5]   McKinsey & Company. (2020). Risk, resilience, and rebalancing in global value chains. https://www.mckinsey.com/business-functions/operations/our-insights/risk-resilience-and-rebalancing-in-global-value-chains.

[6]   Morgan Stanley. (2020). Mapping the new multipolar world order. https://www.morganstanley.com/ideas/coronavirus-global-geopolitics-investing.

[7]   Pisch, F. (2020). Managing Global Production: Theory and Evidence from Just-in-Time Supply Chains. SEPS Discussion Papers 2020–08.

[8]   KPMG's 2020 Global CEO Survey: Special Edition on COVID-19, in Chinese《毕马威2020年全球首席执行官调查：新冠疫情特别版》https://assets.kpmg/content/dam/kpmg/cn/pdf/zh/2020/09/kpmg-2020-ceo-outlook.pdf.

[9]   Shih, W. C. (2020). Global supply chains in a post-pandemic world. *Harvard Business Review*, September–October 2020.

Chapter 5

New Retail in a Post-Covid World

Amy Wong and Allan Chia

Singapore University of Social Sciences, Singapore

The Covid-19 pandemic has impacted all economic sectors, and the retail industry was one of the most affected, as global consumers witnessed the worldwide shutting down of many big names in the brick-and-mortar retail stores such as Abercrombie & Fitch, Bath & Body Works, Robinsons, Victoria's Secret, and JCPenny. At the time of writing, the virus is rapidly spreading in different parts of the world such as India, Russia, the United States, Europe, and Brazil. The dangerous Delta variant has resulted in raging waves of infections in Indonesia, Philippines, Australia, and Malaysia, as lives and livelihoods continue to be affected globally, in every region, every industry, and every aspect of life.

Retailers worldwide are faced with heightened pressure due to changing consumer demand and shopping behaviors, increased health and safety requirements, supply chain disruptions, and labor force shortages, leading to cash flow problems [1]. Physical stores were forced to shutter as countries implemented lockdowns, which compelled shoppers to stay home. As the lockdown prevented front-line retail workers from returning to work, online shopping increased as consumers who were trapped at home started to order more products than ever. Along with the rise in Web 3.0 technology and pandemic-induced social shifts, retailers had to divert their resources to improving their online storefronts and rethinking their e-commerce retail strategy to attract, retain, and engage customers amidst the challenges faced.

To differentiate themselves from competitors, retailers need to understand the changing retail environment, the impact of Covid-19 on retail businesses, and implement innovative solutions to ensure the sustainability of their business models, which will help them stay ahead in today's post-Covid world. This chapter is structured as follows: first, the changing consumer perceptions and behaviors as well as their impact on retail businesses are examined, Next, possible post-pandemic retail scenes are reimagined, while the emergence of new types of retail consumers are presented.

1. Current Retail Challenges

The sudden outbreak of Covid-19 has led to the adoption of lockdown strategies by governments globally, which prevented people from leaving their homes, creating several challenges for retailers. Due to the containment measures in public spaces as well as inside the stores, shoppers have adjusted their purchasing behaviors, with greater tolerance for longer queues and waiting times to enter stores during the pandemic-induced emergency period. The increased governmental regulation for safe distancing has lowered the accessibility to retail store premises, which impacted shoppers' preferred shopping channel, forcing them to switch to other modes of shopping. This was seen in the skyrocketing increase in online grocery shopping during the emergency period, as consumers snapped up all the online shopping delivery slots within minutes of release. In addition, there are continuing concerns regarding the effects of Covid-19 on social distancing, as social isolation can affect consumers' wellbeing, which can cause anxiety, depression, and stress, especially in elderly and vulnerable consumers who find it hard to adjust to the changes [2].

Covid-19 has disrupted the retail industry and impacted brick-and-mortar and online retailers as well as domestic and global retailers in many forms, irrespective of their size, retail format, and product category. Although there may be a temptation for retailers to react to these challenges by implementing aggressive marketing, sales promotions, or operational interventions to increase retail sales and performance, it is vital that retailers take a step back, audit their current brand offerings and retail experience, and explore the possible new opportunities that might arise due to the pandemic. Retailers can start by asking questions related to the latest retail trends, the state of their current consumer lifestyles, consumption patterns, and customer preferences. Retailers can then review and clarify their existing marketing mix strategies, including their product portfolio mix and assortment, pricing options, omnichannel arrangements, and marketing communication tools, while making the effort to adjust these decisions to the post-pandemic retailing scene.

2. Pandemic-Induced Consumer Behaviors

The changes in the external environment have not only affected retailing businesses, but also impacted consumer lifestyles and behaviors. To better understand retail consumer behavior during the pandemic, the current consumer behavior trends in retailing are examined as follows.

2.1 *Panic buying and grocery hoarding*

The Covid-19 pandemic has elevated global anxiety, created a "scarcity effect" and elicited panic buying behavior across the world. During the pandemic, several product categories such as toilet rolls, pasta, and hand sanitizers were hoarded as shoppers engaged in stockpiling in anticipation of a shortfall. For example, surgical masks and hand sanitizers were out of stock in Italy for a few days, while eggs were sold out the day an impending lockdown was announced in Singapore. Although these products were not likely to be needed during the lockdown period, shoppers continued to rush to empty shelves in grocery stores, purchasing brands outside their evoked sets (i.e., products which consumers are likely to purchase), to avoid the possibility of running out of stock. This increased consumer demand due to possible herd mentality and the "fear of missing out" has impacted price elasticities and led to negative impact on the retail supply chain [3].

The hoarding behavior has been examined in a recent study by Leung *et al.* [4], which reported that the spontaneous contagion of public fear fuelled psychological reactions as people took to social media platforms to express their negative views regarding the toilet paper crisis, which further triggered public anxiety and panic. The repeated unavailability of stockout brands and locked down stores altered consumer behaviors, as they began to explore brands outside their preferred choice sets, and might not revert to normality post pandemic [5], increasing the occurrences of switching behaviors.

To curb panic buying, grocery retailers have limited the number of items to be bought per customer, implemented new online priority delivery services and virtual queues, and kept their customers updated on the availability of food. Some retailers operated 24-hour services to stagger demand and introduced contactless curb side delivery to ensure customers' health and safety, while others hired temporary staff from other industries to help in the retail store operations during unexpected peak periods. To manage supply chain disruptions, some retailers have switched to local suppliers where possible, cut their advertising expenditures, and increased food prices.

At FairPrice supermarkets, a chain grocer in Singapore, purchase limits were imposed on staples such as vegetables, rice, toilet paper, and other products, following its neighboring country's announcement on travel restrictions (see Figure 1). As Malaysia is one of the sources of food supply for Singapore, shoppers flocked to the supermarkets to hoard staples, which led to a nation-wide stockout. The retailer, along with local political members, including the Prime Minister, Lee Hsien Loong, provided messages of comfort and assurance that food supplies will continue, and encouraged shoppers to purchase sensibly. The then Minister for Trade and

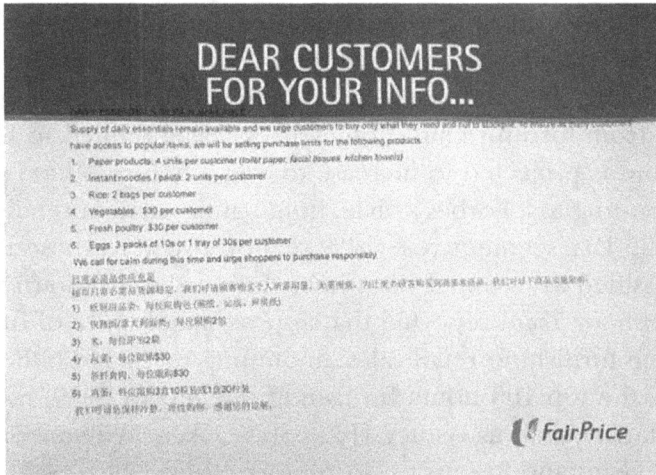

Figure 1. Purchase limits imposed at FairPrice supermarkets in Singapore.

Source: https://www.channelnewsasia.com/singapore/ntuc-fairprice-purchase-limits-toilet-paper-rice-eggs-772846.

Industry, Chan Chun Sing, further clarified that Singapore has plans to manage supplies through stockpiling, local production, and diversification of alternative sources of supplies.

2.2 *The nesting effect*

As consumers stay home during the worldwide imposed quarantine period, many started to invest in home improvement and home decoration products to uplift their work from home spaces. The effect of "home nesting" became a feature of the pandemic as employees spend on home offices, gym equipment, and renovations. Some might prefer self-assemble, mail-to-order furniture that can cosy-proof their living spaces, given the extended duration they spend at home. Others might choose to declutter and reorganize their homes, while some might decide to add a new gym, wellness and massage equipment, or home entertainment system, as a large portion of the workforce shifted to working from home and students moved to online, home-based learning.

The home-furnishing industry has seen an unexpected boom in consumer demand as stay-at-home shoppers opted to refurnish their homes during the pandemic period. In 2020, retail e-commerce revenue from furniture and homeware sales amounted to US$52.6 billion and is projected to increase to over US$61.2 billion in 2025 [6]. According to a Forbes article, home improvement retailers that served the DIY segment rose 14% year-over-year, as these retailers were classified as essential businesses during the lockdown period, while *Furniture Today* reported that approximately 50% of furniture and home furnishing retail sales amounting to US$48 billion were made by the top 100 home furnishing retailers in 2019, including large retailers such as Ashley HomeStore, Ikea, Williams-Sonoma, Mattress Firms and Rooms to Go, among others [7].

Since Covid-19 in 2020, Wayfair, a US-based online furniture store which operates in the US and Europe, has seen a steep rise in its online purchases. Many of their customers were stuck at home, and it was convenient to shop online while continuing to social distance. Housebound customers wanted to make the most of their space because their homes have taken on many roles, such as office, school, gym, and refuge. To help facilitate buyers who have trouble visualizing what a piece of furniture might look like in their homes, a visualization tool, "View in Room" is available on Wayfair's mobile app and permits shoppers to place 3D product images in rooms by using their cameras on their smartphone (see Figure 2). This feature allows shoppers to understand the spatial information and proportion of their rooms as part of an image, and this augmented reality (AR) technology can facilitate mobile shoppers in trying out other décor in a highly customizable manner where they can select their favorite wall and floor color, carpet and curtain design, as well as fabric and accompanying accessories.

2.3 *The rise of digital retailers*

The pandemic has hastened the transition from physical to digital retailing, as e-commerce, m-commerce, and v-commerce orders become an essential part of consumers' everyday lives. Regional

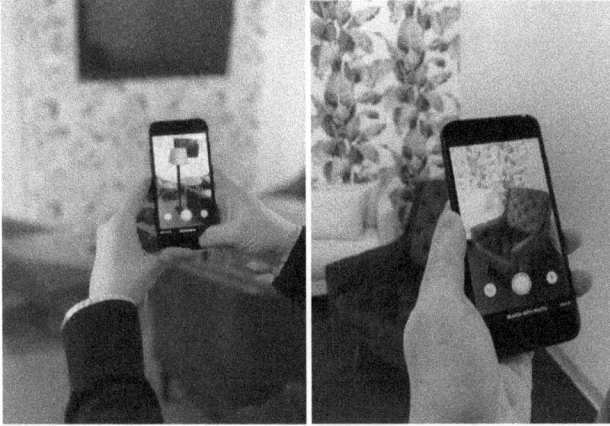

Figure 2. Wayfair "View in Room" AR feature.
Source: https://techcrunch.com/2019/11/13/wayfairs-app-adds-3d-visualization-tools-for-shoppers-including-interactive-photos-a-room-planner/.

online retailers such as Zalando as well as niche retailers such as pet product suppliers Chewy are witnessing a huge growth in market capitalization. These digital retailers were able to benefit from platform economies, scale up and expand their business models to generate increased sales. The surge in digital retailing can be seen in the popularity of Chinese retailers such as Alibaba, JD.com, and Pinduoduo, which delivered 29% of the market capitalization growth in the global retail industry [8].

According to eMarketer, social commerce, which employs social media to promote online transactions, made up 11.6% of e-commerce sales in China in 2020, with an estimated US$242.41 billion [9]. The Chinese major technology giant, Tencent, launched its lite apps know as Mini Programs on WeChat, which allows online retailers and brands to sell their products directly within the WeChat platform. Increasingly, social buyers frequently shop on WeChat live streaming commerce via their mobile devices on-the-go due to its engaging and convenient mode of social buying. WeChat live streaming, a cost-effective live broadcast tool, is mainly used by key opinion leaders (KOL), influencers, and brands to interact with their audience. Brands can set up their own broadcast channel or

PERFECT DIARY
完 美 日 记

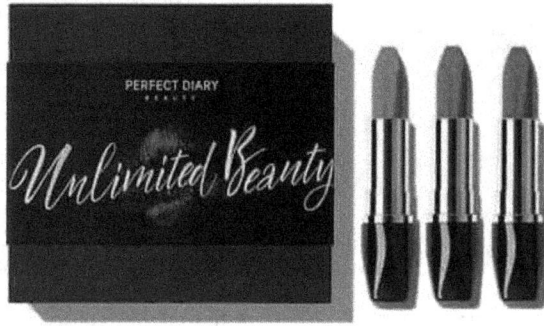

Figure 3.   Perfect Diary, hailed as the "Light of Domestic Goods" in China.
Source: https://marketingtochina.com/perfect-diarys-successful-strategy-on-wechat/.

work with an influencer with a fanbase that is similar to the brand's target audience. Alternatively, live streaming can be conducted through a branded Mini Program, which is available to enterprises. Consumers can use the Mini Program to shop, watch, and interact with sellers.

Perfect Diary, a beauty domestic brand in China established in 2016, is a beauty disruptor that was able to successfully employ a variety of social media platforms to increase its brand awareness and generate high customer engagement, site traffic, and customer purchase (see Figure 3). In 2017, the company engaged a beauty and make-up blogger to deliver a live streaming of make-up demonstration to over a hundred thousand viewers on WeChat Mini Program. Within 150 minutes, the live streaming received 1.7 million likes, achieving an average sales volume increase of over 800%. During the live broadcast, the company's best sellers such as Queen's Day Gift Box and Make-up Brush Set were completely sold out. To date, the bulk of its customers comes from its e-commerce portals, and Perfect Diary has a strong presence on several social media platforms such as Bilibili, Douyin, Little Red Book, Tmall, and Weibo.

2.4 *Return to in-store shopping: Germaphobia and social distancing*

As the lockdowns are lifted, consumers who return to stores will continue to be wary of the virus and its variants, which will not likely be totally eradicated with vaccines. Shoppers who return to in-store shopping will expect higher levels of store cleanliness and hygiene due to germaphobia. Retailers will need to pay attention to safety standards for retail sales and goods delivery. Within the retail store environment, retailers need to focus on their store displays, where surface areas need to be regularly disinfected and wiped down, hand sanitizers and antibacterial wipes need to be provided to all shoppers for disinfecting of shopping carts, and merchandise need to be cling wrapped to prevent direct handling by consumers. In addition, no-touch browsing will become more popular, made possible through the use of portable shopping tablets and touch screens, while in-store food sampling or cosmetic product testing will not be allowed, making it more difficult to promote sensory marketing at the storefront. To ensure the health and safety of frontline retail employees and shoppers, flexible opening hours can be implemented to spread the crowd, as social distancing becomes the norm.

Some government bodies have developed safe management measures and guidelines for retail establishments and lifestyle-related services. In preparation for transition to an endemic state, the Multi-Ministry Taskforce in Singapore has announced a calibrated path for the resumption of economic and social activities with the aim of providing a safe environment for both employees and customers of retailers. These guidelines include safe distancing of at least one meter spacing between groups of up to five persons, clearly demarcated queuing lines for customers at store entrances, masks on and safe entry practices, the need for frequent cleaning and disinfection, as well as the maintenance of proper indoor ventilation and air quality [10].

During Covid-19, AEON Malls, a major Japanese mall operator with 19,288 outlets in Japan, East Asia, and Southeast Asia, invested in measures such as the reduction of customer touchpoints by using digital technology and making changes to facilities so that social distance can be maintained. The disease prevention measures they implemented are based on expert advice and are carried out by all their store employees, working together with customers to create an effective disease prevention system. In February 2021, AEON announced that they would offer their shopping malls in Japan for Covid-19 vaccinations in response to a request by the Japanese government [11].

3. Post-pandemic Retailing

In 2020, retail e-commerce sales worldwide accounted for 18% of all retail sales [12], amounting to US$4.28 trillion, with e-tailing revenue projected to grow to US$5.4 trillion in 2022 [13]. With the advancement of technology and the improved access to affordable mobile broadband connections, online shopping continues to proliferate, especially in fast growing e-retailing markets such as India, Spain, and China. As digital technology continues to disrupt the traditional retailing scene, consumers are progressively embracing the convenience of making purchases via their mobile phones. In Asia, m-commerce, or mobile shopping via a smartphone or a tablet, is gaining popularity, as the percentage of online consumers who have purchased a product via m-commerce continued to rise in 2020, with countries such as Indonesia, Thailand, Philippines, and Malaysia in the lead [14]. Undeniably, technology will continue to disrupt retail businesses, create efficiencies, cut costs, and provide better products and services.

3.1 *Retail leaders vs. laggards*

Despite the challenges of the Covid-19 pandemic, the retail industry has performed generally well compared to other industries such as real estate, air and travel, construction, and oil and gas. Within the retail industry, the gap between retail leaders and laggards has widened, as technologically geared retailers have taken gigantic leaps ahead before the pandemic and managed to gain a strong omnichannel presence. Retail leaders with strong digital footprints such as successful e-commerce companies (i.e., Amazon, Alibaba, JD.com, Pinduoduo, Lowe's, Walmart, and Reliance Industries) continue to thrive, while retail laggards that rely heavily on physical stores with focused product categories such as business apparel and cosmetics continue to lag behind in terms of retail sales. The propelled rise of the retail leaders is reported in a McKinsey study [8], where the top 25 companies that were able to shift to digital saw more than 90% increase in global market capitalization in the industry. These companies comprise four main retail categories, namely home-economy players (i.e., Home Depot), value retailers (i.e., Dollar General), online specialists (i.e., Chewy and Etsy), and platform players (i.e., Shopify). The foundations for their success include the size of the companies, with an average market capitalization of US$122 billion, an average capitalization that is 14.5 times greater than other average retail companies [8].

4. New Consumer Expectations

In a post-pandemic world, consumers will most likely expect more from retailers, hence retailers need to prepare for their customers when they return. Consumers will expect retailer integrity and authenticity, and brands are expected to do the right thing during the pandemic period by placing customer and employee safety and health as their top priorities instead of retail sales or profits. Further, consumers will demand new retailing experiences, and brands can offer fresh and uplifted retailing experiences that can refresh and entertain consumers after a long period of isolation and quarantine, as they transit into a period of post-Covid optimism. Given the increased sensitivity of consumers to safe distancing rules, retailers need to be mindful of crowd management and tight spaces, as retail environment and store atmospherics will play a more critical role. As prolonged safe and social distancing have forced consumers to adapt quickly to online platforms such as e-commerce, m-commerce, v-commerce, and s-commerce (i.e., social commerce) sites as well as live selling on social media platforms, retailers need to ride on the digital disruption wave and continue to adapt to the new hierarchy of needs of the re-emerging online audience.

To survive the pandemic, retailers need to anticipate a post-pandemic retail scene, reimagine the store of the future, and commence the digital transformation process to align to the new reality. Retailers should respond to this digital opportunity by capitalizing on technology as an enabler of better customer service and greater operational competencies across all parts of the retail ecosystem. Some of the retail strategies that retailers can consider are discussed in what follows.

4.1 *The retail ecosystem*

The retail ecosystem, which consists of the network of suppliers, partners, and channel members, can be orchestrated to support the retailer's business model to attain customer lifetime value maximization. The entire retail ecosystem needs to adopt an agile and responsive approach to understanding customer needs, providing value-added products, services, and solutions, delivering customer satisfaction, and achieving customer loyalty, leading to long-term relationship profitability. To accomplish this, the main actor (i.e., the retailer) needs to build a collaborative culture, break free of functional and organizational boundaries, embrace state-of-the-art technology, and create new opportunities in the online-to-offline (O2O) connected retail scene. Examples of dominant retail ecosystems include the big four technology companies such as Apple, Amazon, Facebook, and Google. These technology giants are investing more in retailer solutions such as voice-based shopping solutions (i.e., Amazon's Alexa), facial recognition equipment in stores (i.e., Amazon Go), and food ordering features in mobile apps (i.e., Google).

Increasingly, retail ecosystems are gaining a strong foothold in Asia, as the interconnected players such as retailers, consumers, and stakeholders (i.e., financial and logistic partners, channel members, suppliers, marketing intermediaries) participate in different forms, across various stages of growth. In Asia, huge technological players such as Tencent have built up an open ecosystem, providing customers with a one-stop shop such as e-commerce, m-commerce, and

One-stop shop for shoppers   **Solutions for retail partners**

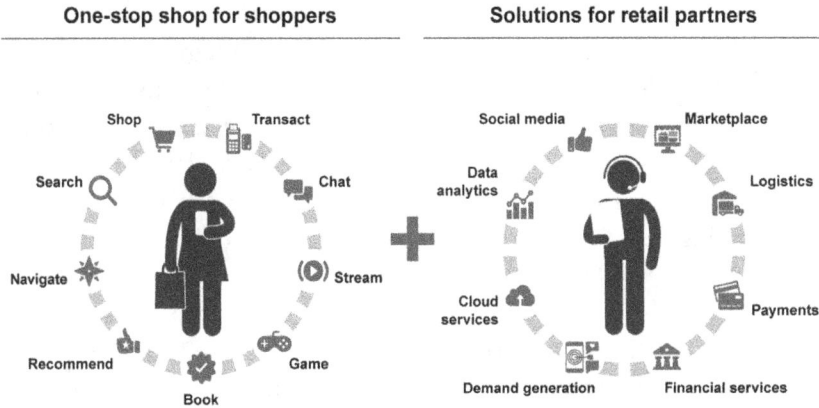

Figure 4.   Players in the retail ecosystem.

Source: Bain & Company, https://www.bain.com/insights/the-future-of-retailing-asias-retail-ecosystems-report/.

s-commerce (i.e., social commerce) options and integrated services, chat, live streaming, gaming, online booking for different products and services (i.e., ride-hailing, laundry, pet sitting, home cleaning, food delivery), and payments in a single platform or app. Tencent's WeChat has one billion subscribers, who are transforming the retail experience in partnership with JD.com, providing one-stop shop solutions for shoppers and retail partners. As part of Tencent's retail ecosystem, the different partners can tap into Tencent's marketplace, social media channels, data analytics capabilities, cloud services, financial services, logistics, demand generation, payment model, and online marketplace [15]. An ecosystem can deliver great benefits for shoppers and partners alike, providing the players with added capacity to reinvest and access the competitive advantages of the ecosystem (see Figure 4).

4.2 *From companies to platforms*

Companies that benefitted from platform economies were able to scale up and expand their business models to generate returns through business diversification and adaptability. As part of a platform economy, companies can offer their products and services through open platforms, access the consumer resources and capabilities of others within the platform, and integrate their operations, product and service offerings, and contributions with other platform players, such as suppliers and customers. Indeed, a well-functioning platform can attract committed developers and supportive customers, and such a network effect can elevate the brand value, performance, and overall sales of the participating companies.

According to a Forbes article on platform businesses, several guidelines can boost platform success [16]. To benefit from platform economies, retailers can concentrate on their strategic core and bundle their offerings around user value and brand experience. As retailers need to depend on the success of other players in platform economies, they need to give other players a chance to contribute to the refinement of their business requirements to ensure synergy among platform partners. By offering their products and services through application programming interfaces (APIs), a connection between computers or between computer programs, retailers can convert their valuable user data and consumer demographic information into insights for themselves and their platform partners.

During the pandemic, a retailer e-commerce platform provider, GoDaddy, responded to the needs of new to intermediate online retailers by making their website and some of its marketing support access-free. The platform offers easy to customize and optimize templates for m-commerce and provides features such as search engine optimization (SEO) to help improve website traffic quality and quantity. Other features include online promotion banners, integration with local advertising in Google, Facebook, and Instagram, advanced data analytics, as well as payment and shipping tools designed to support small retailers.

4.3 *The phygital retail environment*

Along with the rise in disruptive technology, the retail environment, consisting of online and offline environments, has merged into a phygital environment that encapsulates the best aspects of both spaces. A phygital environment taps on the strengths of online retailing such as immediacy, immersion, and speed, as well as the opportunity for interaction and the evoking of all five senses in physical retailing. An omnichannel retailing strategy can effectively connect shoppers' O2O experiences, allowing them to interchange between these two phases easily, creating intensified interactions that can boost brand awareness and affinity.

As the lockdown eases, it is important that retailers recognize the seamless relationship between the two O2O channels, which can help equip them to offer a phygital retailing experience. As consumers reassess their shopping habits, they might discover new benefits that they were unfamiliar with pre-pandemic. Elderly consumers might have switched to online retailing during the pandemic and discovered the safety of home-deliveries and cashless payments. Post pandemic, these consumers might continue with show rooming, where the physical store is used as a showroom for feeling and trying out the product, but the actual purchase is made online for its convenience. On the other hand, younger consumers who are used to online shopping might yearn for physical interactions with family and friends, and these consumers might prefer to shop at the brick-and-mortar stores after web rooming or engaging in prior online product review research. Post pandemic, consumers might continue to seek digital retailing while shopping in-store, as they use their mobile phones to search for price comparisons, promotions, ratings, reviews, and information on the product.

Amazon Fresh is a good example of phygital as it offers a blended customer experience where both the physical and digital coexist. It opened its first UK store in London in 2021. The store concept allows consumers to shop and leave without scanning items or queuing to pay. The Amazon app is used to bring the physical and digital experience together. Customers enter by scanning a QR code generated by the app, and cameras and sensors track what items they are selecting in the store, placing them in a virtual cart. After consumers leave the shop, they are charged through their Amazon account and emailed the receipt. There are no queues and this phygital model also provides Amazon with useful purchase data to analyze and inform decision-makers on future marketing strategies, both online and offline.

4.4 *Transition to digital retailing*

The digital grocery experience is currently faced with high market demand, as consumers constantly find it hard to secure a delivery time slot, and product inventory continues to fluctuate, leading to much longer than usual waiting times. The scarcity of orders made the delivery service even more desirable to consumers, as consumer competition for orders prevails. This further accelerated the digital disruption of grocery, where grocers start charging for packing fee and small order service fee, introducing priority delivery slots for vulnerable consumers, or prioritizing delivery timings for different groups of customers.

When stores are finally allowed to reopen, retailers need to transit to the "new normal." Innovative retail technology such as interactive shop windows, self-service, multi-users touchscreens, digital signages, virtual shopping carts, as well as mobile payments can be harnessed in the day-to-day retail operations to facilitate contactless and safe shopping. For better customer engagement in physical stores, transparent displays using AR can offer a futuristic approach to experiencing a product. This technology can be applied on delicate luxury products such as jewelry or watches. Similarly, clothing or accessory retailers can adopt virtual fitting rooms for ease of trying out apparels of different colors and styles, or handbags of different shapes and sizes. Conversely, online retailers can also implement retail technologies such as virtual reality (VR) stores and create AR apps for Apple, Android, and Window interfaces that customers can download and browse on-the-go.

Zara was one of the largest clothing retailers to introduce AR displays in their stores. Originally intended to lure millennials, these AR displays in pandemic times enable shoppers to select and try clothing items with minimal physical contact. The AR features allow shoppers to view models wearing selected looks from its range of clothes. With the use of a mobile phone, they can hold it up to a sensor within a store or designated shop windows and click through to buy the clothes. Zara's AR technology also enables models to pop up "virtually" on packages of online purchases that have been delivered, which can then display alternative outfits for customers to choose from.

4.5 *Big data, safe data, and dirty data*

During the pandemic, governmental regulations with regards to quarantine order and contact tracing have led to consumers' higher acceptance of body scanning surveillance measures, temperature taking devices, GPS tracking, or facial recognition [5]. Over the prolonged pandemic period, consumers might have gotten used to such invasive technologies and might be more willing to disclose their personal information for health and safety purposes. Although consumer privacy and personal information disclosure will always remain a concern post-pandemic, retailers can experiment with big data analytics at every stage of the retail process, from forecasting demand for products, to optimizing product prices, and even to identifying likely products that customers are interested in.

For many years, retailers have benefited from structured (i.e., clean) data collected via their customer database system or through their store loyalty programs, where direct mails and customized marketing messages have been communicated to their target shoppers as part of their direct marketing efforts. Only recently, retailers have begun paying attention to unstructured (i.e., dirty) data, comprising inaccurate, incomplete, inconsistent, and duplicate datasets that are freely available in social media platforms, customer online feedback, recorded store or product videos, and locational GPS data. By prioritizing investments in advanced data analytics and customer personalization across multiple channels, retailers can combine different interactive retail technologies to deliver an innovative and rich customer experience.

Advancement in technology has allowed retailers to use both structured and unstructured data to provide valuable insights that can help them make informed decisions in real time, based upon trending customer needs. Retailers can collect big data via consumers' interconnected smart devices which can leave digital traces, allowing them to follow the customer journeys and paths digitally. Capitalizing on social media data, which consists of unstructured data such as tweets, videos, audio, photos, and location data, retailers can predict real-time trends and consumer sentiments about their products and services. One excellent example is Target, a general merchandise retailer that sells products through its stores and digital channels, which garnered national attention when it managed to use big data and predictive analytics to predict a teen's pregnancy before her family found out.

5. The Emergence of a New Consumer

The profound changes brought about by the Covid-19 outbreak have impacted consumer lifestyles and behaviors, leading to the emergence of new types of retail consumers, presented as follows.

5.1 *The tech-savvy consumer*

The worldwide lockdowns have spurred the launch of several online players, as existing niche companies, online platforms, and leading retailers experience market-cap growth, exacerbated mainly by the rise of the tech-savvy consumer. These digital age consumers enjoy enhanced hedonism and derive pleasure from on-demand, social-driven, entertaining shopping experiences. The tech-savvy consumer will continue to seek innovative retail technologies such as extended reality (XR), comprising VR, AR, mixed-reality (MR), as well as artificial intelligence (AI)-powered chatbots that can improve the authenticity and trustworthiness of the shopping experience.

5.2 *The prudent consumer*

The unusual circumstances of the pandemic have led to several global retrenchments, unprecedented job losses, and early retirement in industries such as airline, travel, hospitality, retailing, food and beverage, as well as real estate, and this is made worse with the displacement of job roles due to technology and automation. As a result, many affected households have become extra careful and value-oriented, concentrating their household consumption decisions on things that are needful. Leading value retailers such as Costco, Daiso, TJX, Ikea, and Dollar General were able to capitalize on this trend to deliver products and services that get the job done.

5.3 *The responsible consumer*

The shift in mindset toward socially responsible behavior has heightened during the pandemic period. The scarcity of sanitizers and surgical masks during the early pandemic period have led to several innovative business practices geared toward socially responsible initiatives such as traditional spirits and alcohol producers reconfiguring their production to hand sanitizers and giving it away for free to hospital workers and vulnerable people. Traditional tailors and stay-home-mums have come together to hand sew face masks in replacement of surgical masks and distributing them to younger children, elderly, or frontline workers. Luxury retailers such as Burberry and Prada have reconfigured their factories to produce medical garments, while Dyson has produced ventilators for hospital patients [5]. Several retailers, large and small, have initiated socially responsible practices to care for the society, for example, donating to hospitals or charities, or sending care packs to frontline workers.

5.4 *The resilient consumer*

The pandemic-induced changes such as health fears, consumer confidence, economic concerns, and new live-at-work arrangements have clearly impacted consumer lifestyles and buying behavior. Although the pandemic forces consumers to remain indoors, consumers continue to stay fully occupied, using this prolonged confinement period to redecorate their homes, take up a new hobby, embrace new beauty routines, adopt new clothing styles, adjust to online zoom fitness classes, as well as care for their families, friends, and pets. The stress of the pandemic due to unemployment and inflation has brought about greater emphasis on consumer wellbeing, with topics such as mindfulness, mental, emotional, and physical wellbeing being discussed more openly. These new consumer habits will most likely endure beyond the pandemic period, leading to a permanent change in what consumers seek and value in the long run, as the resilient consumer emerges as someone who might be financially constrained, tech-savvy, highly selective, and adaptable to new pressures, realities, and opportunities.

6. Conclusion

The Covid-19 pandemic has altered consumer perceptions, lifestyles, and behavior. As the world navigates out of the pandemic, retailers are faced with the challenges of attracting, retaining, and managing consumers with changed and renewed mindsets and perspectives in the post-pandemic environment. The chapter examined the changing consumer perceptions and behavior including panic buying, the nesting effect, digital retailing, germaphobia, and social distancing as well as their impact on retail businesses. The possible post-pandemic retail scenes, exacerbated by new consumer expectations, are reimagined. This includes the emergence of retail ecosystems, retail platforms, phygital, and digital retailing as well as big data. Finally, the new types of retail consumers, namely the tech-savvy, prudent, responsible, and resilient consumers are described. The Covid-19 outbreak may provide an opportunity for retailers who are pre-emptive, innovative, creative, and agile enough to ride along the waves of destruction and disruption, as they challenge their existing systems and embrace transformation wholeheartedly, as many of their successful predecessors have done so.

References

[1] Goldberg, J. (2020). The impact of Covid-19 on U.S. brands and retailers. *Forbes*. https://www.forbes.com/sites/jasongoldberg/2020/03/29/the-impact-of-covid-19-on-us-brands-and-retailers/?sh=7d63b3df1452.

[2] Torales, J., O'Higgins, M., Castaldelli-Maia, J. M., and Ventriglio, A. (2020). The outbreak of COVID-19 coronavirus and its impact on global mental health. *International Journal of Social Psychiatry*, **66**(4), 317–320.

[3] Ivanov, D. (2020). Predicting the impacts of epidemic outbreaks on global supply chains: A simulation-based analysis on the coronavirus outbreak (COVID-19. SARS-CoV-2) case. *Transportation Research Part E: Logistics and Transportation Review*, **136**, 101922.

[4] Leung, J., Chung, J. Y. C., Tisdale, C., Chiu, V., Lim, C. C. W., and Chang, G. (2021). Anxiety and panic buying behaviour during COVID-19 pandemic — A qualitative analysis of toilet paper hoarding contents on Twitter. *International Journal of Environmental Research and Public Health*, **18**(3), 1127.

[5] Pantano, E., Pizzi, G., Scarpi, D., and Dennis, C. (2020). Competing during a pandemic? Retailers' ups and downs during the Covid-19 outbreak. *Journal of Business Research*, **116**, 209–213.

[6] Statista Research Department. (2021). Furniture and homeware e-commerce revenue in the United States from 2017 to 2025. *Statista*.

[7] Danziger, P. N. (2021). Retailers are losing. Only the big and virtual will survive. *Forbes*. https://www.forbes.com/sites/pamdanziger/2021/03/28/independent-home-furnishings-retailers-are-losing-only-the-strong-and-virtual-will-survive/?sh=6fae40fe4484.

[8] Bradley, C., Kohli, S., Kuijpers, D., and Smith, T. R. (2021). Why retail outperformers are pulling ahead, McKinsey & Company. https://www.mckinsey.com/industries/consumer-packaged-goods/our-insights/why-retail-outperformers-are-pulling-ahead.

[9] Kats, R. (2020). In China, social commerce makes up 11.6% of retail ecommerce sales. eMarketer insider intelligence. https://www.emarketer.com/content/china-social-commerce-makes-up-11-6-of-retail-ecommerce-sales.

[10] Singapore Tourism Board. (2021). Safe management measures for retail establishments. https://www.stb.gov.sg/content/stb/en/home-pages/advisory-for-retail-establishments.html.

[11] Reuters. (2021). Japan's Aeon says to offer shopping malls nation-wide for COVID-19 vaccinations. 12 February. https://www.reuters.com/article/us-health-coronavirus-japan-aeon-idUSKBN2AC0W0.

[12] Coppola, D. (2021). Worldwide e-commerce share of retail sales 2015–2024. *Statista*.

[13] Sabanoglu, T. (2021a). Global retail e-commerce sales 2014–2024. *Statista*.

[14] Sabanoglu, T. (2021b). Mobile commerce reach in selected countries 2020. *Statista*.

[15] Sanders, M., Parekh, K., Kang, H., Kamel, M. A., and Cheng, J. (2018). The future of retail: Asia's ecosystems: Asia's retail sales boom has given rise to a new concept with massive implications. Report, Bain & Company. https://www.bain.com/insights/the-future-of-retailing-asias-retail-ecosystems-report/.

[16] McKendrick, J. (2019). Once they were companies, now they are platform businesses. *Forbes*. https://www.forbes.com/sites/joemckendrick/2019/01/23/once-they-were-companies-now-they-are-platform-businesses/?sh=f3c68ff27736.

Chapter 6

Evolution of China's Crisis Management: A Comparison of Covid-19 and SARS

Chen Gang

East Asian Institute, National University of Singapore, Singapore

Two months after the Chinese Communist Party (CCP) convened its Fourth Plenum that emphasized modernization of China's governance capacity, a novel coronavirus (Covid-19) outbreak in the likes of SARS (Severe Acute Respiratory Syndrome) erupted in the central Chinese city of Wuhan in December 2019 (Appendix), which spread like wildfire to other provinces and abroad in the beginning of 2020, causing massive cases of death and triggering panic across the country and the world. On 30 January 2020, the World Health Organization (WHO) declared Covid-19 a global health emergency, a declaration accorded for extremely dangerous pandemics such as Ebola and Swine Flu (H1N1 virus).

Covid-19 triggered another public health emergency after SARS that tested the Chinese leadership's crisis management capacity. The CCP has drawn lessons from the SARS outbreak 17 years earlier: the Hu Jintao–Wen Jiabao leadership, right in their first year in power, sacked incompetent senior officials for their covering up and mishandling of the SARS outbreak. Strict quarantines and travel restrictions, together with subsequent transparent reporting and communication systems, had helped the Hu–Wen Administration pass the first stress test and consolidate power at home. Covid-19 broke out in the middle of Xi Jinping's second term as paramount leader, and similarly, through large-scale lockdown measures and massive medical support, China finally brought down the number of cases significantly within its border. Nevertheless, although China's response to Covid-19 was largely based on lessons and experiences learned during the SARS period, the local government still made similar mistakes by suppressing vital information in the early days of the pandemic. Moreover, there were significant differences between the two crisis managements in terms of top leaders' roles, reshuffling of local officials, participation of the military forces, development of vaccines, and relevant laws and regulations relating the two responses. This particular study, through delving into the key consistencies and variations in China's handling of SARS and Covid-19, reveals what political factors are strongly correlated with the evolution of the CCP's crisis management in the reform era, with a focus on the comparison of Xi Jinping and Hu Jintao's responses to the two pandemics and on the institutional environments where the crises were managed.

1. Initial Government Reactions

Covid-19, which was initially labeled as 2019-nCoV, was first detected in Wuhan in December 2019. The human-to-human transmission of the virus was confirmed on 20 January 2020 (Appendix) [1]. Covid-19 is caused by a betacoronavirus, like the Middle East Respiratory Syndrome (MERS) and SARS, all of which may have their origins in bats [2]. China adopted anti-SARS measures as the natural policy response to the H1N1 outbreak in 2009 and to the coronavirus-affected areas in Wuhan in 2020.

While the SARS epidemic started in southern China's Guangdong province, the coronavirus erupted in Wuhan city, a densely populated megacity with a population of more than 11 million and right at the nexus of China's transportation webs. Wuhan has a nickname of *jiu sheng tong qu* (九省通衢), which literally translates as "the main thoroughfare of nine provinces." On land, in addition to conventional railway networks, Wuhan is one of the main stops on two of the main long-haul, high-speed railway lines: Beijing–Guangzhou (from north to south) and Shanghai–Chengdu (from east to west). In the air, Wuhan Tianhe International Airport is the only airport in central China to have direct flights to five different continents. At sea, Wuhan is a bustling river port along the Yangtze River that connects the coastal area with the hinterland.

Wuhan's pivotal location in China's terrain and China's modernization of transport and logistical networks in recent years have significantly increased the risks and difficulties in the government's responses to the lethal coronavirus. In 2003, there was no high-speed railway, and the number of people traveling by air and across borders was only a fraction of today's scale. For example, about 68,000 railway passengers left Wuhan on the first day of the Spring Festival in 2003 while in 2020, the figure surged by about four times to 270,000, a factor for the rapid spread of the virus. On 20 January 2020, only four provinces including Hubei reported of confirmed cases; by 24 January, the number increased to 30 out 31 provinces. It took months for SARS to transmit to 26 provinces in 2002/2003.

By 21 February 2020, China updated the total number of infected cases to 75,567, with 2,239 deaths, both of which were much higher than the figures during SARS, which stood at 5,327 and 349, respectively, for mainland China. The first death from the Wuhan virus was reported on 11 January 2020 in Wuhan. According to WHO data, most of the infected cases were found in China.

The Chinese government reported on the coronavirus to WHO on 31 December 2019, less than a month from the detection of the virus, which was much quicker than the case for SARS. On 12 January 2020, China shared the genetic sequence of the novel coronavirus with the international research community and in public databases such as GenBank, the US NIH (National Institutes of Health) genetic sequence database.

On 26 January 2020, a leading small group (LSG) on the prevention and control of the outbreak of new pneumonia caused by the novel coronavirus was established at the central government level led by Premier Li Keqiang (the first leading group he is leading) and with Politburo Standing Committee member Wang Huning as the deputy leader. Having served as an adviser to three Chinese presidents, namely, Jiang Zemin, Hu Jintao, and Xi Jinping, Wang Huning is now the top party official in charge of ideology, propaganda, and party organization [3].

Li and Wang's roles in the LSG, however, do not necessarily mean that Chinese President Xi Jinping is outside of the top decision-making on anti-epidemic work. On 28 January 2020, Xi met the executive director of WHO, Dr Tedros Adhanom Ghebreyesus, and told him that he "personally directed" the government's response to the outbreak [4]. Xi presided over two top-level CCP Politburo Standing Committee meetings on 3 February and 12 February, both of which were shown at length on Chinese television. Xi declared a "people's war" and "total war" on the coronavirus outbreak, saying "the success of the nationwide response hinges on Hubei province, and the success of Hubei's response hinges on Wuhan city" [5].

Local governments also took a number of draconian measures. An unprecedented lockdown was imposed on Wuhan city. Since 10 a.m. in the morning of 23 January (local time), all public transport including buses, trains, subways, and ferries were shut down in the city. Major roads linking Wuhan were also blocked. More than a dozen cities (located mostly in Hubei province) took similar measures on public transport. By 25 January 2020, 30 out of 31 provinces in China had activated the highest-level emergency response for public health (Level I). Tibet activated the second highest level emergency (Level II) on 27 January 2020.

According to the National Master Plan for Responding to Public Emergencies (国家突发公共事件总体应急预案) enacted in 2006 by the State Council, public emergency events in China can be classified into four categories: public health emergencies, natural disasters, accidents, and emergencies threatening public security [6]. The State Council has set up a four-level response system on all emergencies based on their severity and controllability, namely, Level I (most severe, red-coded), Level II (very severe, orange-coded), Level III (severe, yellow-coded), and Level IV (general, blue-coded). According to the National Plan for Responding to Public Health Emergencies (国家突发公共卫生事件应急预案), which was also enacted in 2006, the spread of any contagious SARS-like virus or human infection from avian flu, requires the government to immediately activate Level I emergency response [7]. Any unidentified epidemic that involves cases in multiple provinces also deserves Level I response [7].

The outbreak raises several serious concerns about China's crisis management capability, especially in the public health realm. Level I responses were not triggered in time, which came late between 23 and 25 January. Despite the framework for national emergency responses that was put in place by the State Council after SARS, the initial reporting and assessment of the epidemic, as well as the coordination of government departments, proved to be inadequate.

Specially, the Regulation on Handling Public Health Emergencies in May 2003, Law on the Prevention and Control of Infectious Diseases in 2004 to clarify the responsibility of local government and health authorities in infectious disease surveillance and reporting, and regulations on contingency plans during a public crisis for central ministries and local governments in 2006 and 2011 apparently did not measure up. Information disclosure was still not swift enough for Covid-19. The delay in information disclosure could be a result of an ineffective coordination between the Wuhan municipal government and other government departments.

2. Political Changes after the Outbreak

Like other major disasters and emergency events, the outbreak had immediate impact on party official reshuffling, while the ripple effects may have long-term influence on institutional building and personnel arrangement in Chinese politics. During the public outrage over officials' cover-up of SARS outbreak in 2003, the top leadership sacked both Beijing Mayor Meng Xuenong and Minister of Health Zhang Wenkang, while in the case of Covid-19, Beijing removed Hubei Provincial Party Secretary Jiang Chaoliang and Wuhan Municipal Party Secretary Ma Guoqiang over "botched" outbreak response [8]. In contrast to Beijing's punishment during SARS that was targeted at administrative chiefs, the initial purge this time was aimed at party chiefs who generally have a final say in local affairs and thus are more accountable for poor governance.

Shanghai Mayor Ying Yong, 61, a close ally of Xi Jinping, became the new party boss of Hubei province, while Wang Zhonglin, 57, party secretary of Jinan, the capital city of the eastern province of Shandong, was appointed party secretary of Wuhan city [8]. Both Ying and Wang have work experience in the political and legal system (政法系统) that includes police and other law enforcement departments.

Ying was police chief of Shaoxing city in Zhejiang province and chief of the Zhejiang provincial court and Shanghai municipal court, while Wang worked for local police and procuratorate departments in Shandong province [9]. Xi Jinping himself had worked in both Zhejiang province and Shanghai municipality before joining the Politburo Standing Committee in 2007.

Chen Yixin, secretary-general of the Commission for Political and Legal Affairs of the CCP Central Committee, was appointed deputy head of a central government group to guide epidemic control work in Hubei province. Chen was former deputy Party chief of Hubei province and former leading official of Wuhan before he was transferred to the Commission for Political and Legal Affairs in Beijing [10]. As they have work experience in the political and legal system, the appointment of Ying, Wang, and Chen shows Beijing's strong political will to control the epidemic through draconian social management approaches, including strict quarantine, information control, and regulation of social and economic activities.

Various cities near Wuhan also stepped up quarantine efforts. The small center of Wuxue, on 15 February, announced that with the exception of people working to contain the epidemic, anyone seen walking along the streets would be sent to a stadium for "study sessions" [11]. Beijing also appointed two senior firefighting commanders to the Ministry of Emergency Management's leading group — Xu Ping, head of the ministry's Forest Fire Bureau, and Qiong Se, director of its Fire and Rescue Bureau. Xu was a general from the People's Armed Police, while Qiong Se had previously worked for the local police in Zhejiang province and the Ministry of Public Security in Beijing.

The Chinese government will generally set up *ad hoc* inter-agency panels in the aftermath of catastrophic disasters, which are normally built on the existing state apparatus responding to public emergencies. During the 8.0-magnitude Sichuan earthquake in 2008, the central government set up the Earthquake Relief Headquarters, while during the 2010 Yangtze River floods, the State Flood Control and Drought Relief Headquarters commanded the disaster relief campaign [12].

The central government this time established the LSG on the prevention and control of the outbreak of new pneumonia caused by the novel coronavirus (中央应对新冠肺炎疫情工作领导小组), with Premier Li Keqiang and Wang Huning, a Politburo Standing Committee member, as the respective chief and deputy chief. Since Wang is in charge of party affairs instead of state affairs, his role in the LSG is to ensure the party's control of the state apparatus in the fight against the epidemic.

Another two *ad hoc* institutions were respectively set up at the central and local levels to ensure the supervision and implementation of directives from Beijing. Vice Premier Sun Chunlan headed the central government group to guide epidemic control work in Hubei province (中央赴湖北指导组), which supervised the local government's work against coronavirus, while the Hubei party secretary and governor led epidemic control headquarters in Hubei province (湖北省新型冠状病毒感染肺炎疫情防控指挥部), which directly organized epidemic control work and implemented central directives on the frontline (Table 1).

Although both the LSG and the central government group to guide epidemic control work were headed by leaders from the State Council (Premier Li Keqiang and Vice Premier Sun Chunlan, respectively), Xi Jinping, the paramount leader, has been playing a vital role in commanding the prevention and control work of the outbreak, indicating the Party's strengthened grip over state apparatus since the administrative reform in 2018.[i] According to a report from China's

---

[i] For details of this reform, please refer to Reference [13].

Table 1.   Chinese government's commanding system of novel coronavirus control work.

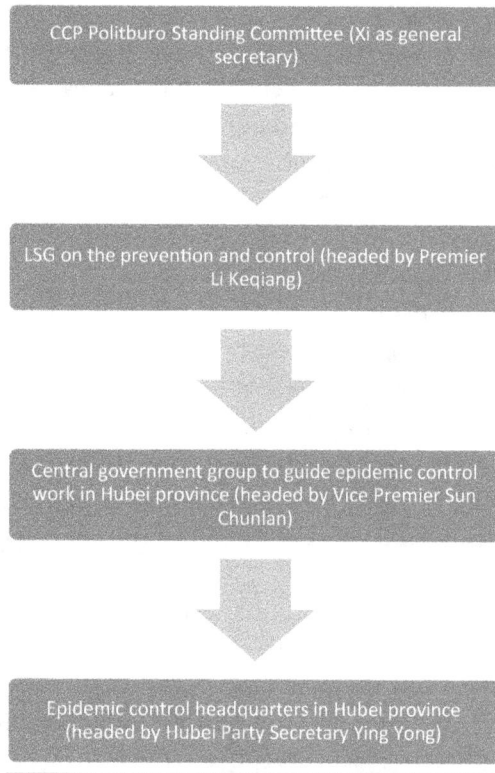

CCP Politburo Standing Committee (Xi as general secretary)

↓

LSG on the prevention and control (headed by Premier Li Keqiang)

↓

Central government group to guide epidemic control work in Hubei province (headed by Vice Premier Sun Chunlan)

↓

Epidemic control headquarters in Hubei province (headed by Hubei Party Secretary Ying Yong)

Source: Compiled by the author.

official *Xinhua News Agency,* entrusted by Xi, Vice Premier Sun Chunlan inspected a newly delivered hospital in Wuhan [14], indicating Xi's prerogative in directing the central government group on epidemic work. In meeting with Dr Tedros Adhanom Ghebreyesus, WHO director general, in Beijing on 28 January, Xi said he was "personally commanding" the response to the outbreak [15].

The death of Dr Li Wenliang, a whistleblower, almost turned the issue into a public confidence crisis for Beijing in February. Li, a 34-year-old ophthalmologist, was one of the eight whistle-blowers disciplined by the police in early January for "rumor mongering" after he posted a message on a closed online WeChat group about a number of "SARS-like" cases at his hospital. He contracted the infection from treating patients, and his death transformed him into an icon [16]. The National Supervisory Commission, the top anti-corruption state agency, sent an inspection group to Wuhan to thoroughly investigate issues related to Li, signaling how seriously it was taking public anger over the handling of the outbreak.

3. Central vs. Local

The resilience to catastrophes is fundamentally local, which involves the strengths of the local government and community to prepare for, respond to, and recover from disasters. As such, an axiomatic principle is that the remedy in terms of protection and relief must be applied at the grass-roots level of local communities and administrations [17]. Local capacity-building and solutions to disaster management therefore are essential for effective risk management, disaster responses, and recovery efforts; in today's interconnected and bureaucracy-laden crisis management field, however, local disaster resilience is often constrained by limited fiscal and human resources, disengaged citizens, and conflicting local government priorities [18].

Local authorities since the early 1990s have been allocated greater political and fiscal autonomy in dealing with local issues that include public emergency jobs. Nevertheless, in a still centralized one-party political system, local apparatus is not prepared to play an independent role in most response and recovery actions. As in other policy realms, China's public health emergency management, to a large extent, is still vertically organized.

Local officials could only play a very passive role in control, relief and recover, often finding themselves being excluded from the process of decision-making, organization, and coordination. However, limited power does not necessarily come with limited responsibilities. In a centralized system of cadre promotion, local officials are accountable for local crisis management results, bearing unavoidable responsibilities which may add risks to their political careers.

For many people in China, Dr Li Wenliang's death offered a release of pent-up anger and frustration with how the government mishandled the situation with the withholding of information and silencing of whistle-blowers [19]. It indicated that the government had not learned lessons from previous crises, such as SARS 17 years ago, and continued to quash online criticism and investigative reports that provide vital information.

In response to the widespread outcry, the CCP's bimonthly journal *Qiushi* on 15 February published an internal speech given by Xi on 3 February, instructing the Politburo Standing Committee to tackle the outbreak of the coronavirus, almost 2 weeks before the Chinese authorities announced that there had been human-to-human transmission of the disease [11].

In his speech on 3 February, Xi also accused local officials of not carrying out edicts from the central government, vowing to punish incompetent officials. "I issued demands during a Politburo Standing Committee meeting on January 7 for work to contain the outbreak. On January 20, I gave special instructions about the work to prevent and control the outbreak and I have said we have to pay high attention to it," he said [11].

In that speech, Xi said that the outbreak not only endangers the health of the Chinese people but also jeopardizes the country's economic and social stability — even its Open Door Policy. The speech, published by journal *Qiushi* 12 days after its delivery, was also featured on state television and other official mouthpieces, showing Xi's active engagement in handling the crisis from an early date, and that local government officials should be held accountable for the dereliction of duty.

Xi and his team are facing a severe test with the Wuhan coronavirus. The outbreak happened at a time when China is to achieve its first centenary goal of becoming a full *Xiaokang* (moderately well-off) society before 2021, as denoted by the doubling of the 2010 per capita GDP. The contagious coronavirus is not only challenging the fulfillment of the government's ambitious economic blueprint, but also testing Xi's plan on governance capacity building, a highlight at the Fourth Plenum. In China's 4,000-year-long history and modern development, disaster politics has always been the ultimate test for the top leadership in power.

China's annual parliamentary meetings, scheduled for early March 2020, were postponed because of the Covid-19 outbreak.

The parliamentary sessions of the National People's Congress (NPC) and the Chinese People's Political Consultative Conference (CPPCC) in every March, commonly known as the *lianghui* (literally the "two meetings"), constitute one of the most important events on China's annual political agenda and an important forum for debates on socioeconomic issues and approval of laws, policies, budget, and government report. The delay will slow down China's law-making process, as well as the State Council's work relating to budgeting and economic planning.

4. Military Forces in China's Crisis Management

Like many other countries, the Chinese leadership often calls upon its armed forces to assist with large-scale rescue and relief operations in times of natural catastrophes. The frequency, scale, and types of rescue and relief works that the People's Liberation Army (PLA) has conducted are seldom matched by military forces elsewhere. In recent years, when the PLA was shifting its strategic focus to non-traditional security issues (*feichuantong anquan wenti*), its tasks in domestic rescue and relief activities became even more important.

Since the PLA has its own autonomous administrative and operation process, central and local government officials often have an awkward relationship with the PLA in the crisis management system where the PLA only obeys orders from the Central Military Commission (CMC) rather than administrative leaders. Neither the LSG on the prevention and control of the outbreak nor the central government group to guide epidemic control work could directly command the PLA in handling the epidemic.

In China's unique system of "Party commanding the Gun" (*dang zhihui qiang*), the Party's CMC is in full command of PLA affairs, with only the Party's general secretary sitting in as commander-in-chief and assisted by top generals. As compared to Hu Jintao, Xi's predecessor, who left its operation largely to the PLA, Xi managed to consolidate his power in the military through daunting anti-corruption investigations. Xi has repeatedly emphasized the importance of the PLA's absolute loyalty and firm faith in the Party leadership, reiterating the party's supremacy over the PLA on various occasions. Xi's dominance over the PLA was evident during the second Sichuan Earthquake in Ya'an in 2013, when the PLA troops were immediately deployed to disaster-stricken areas at the request of the State Council.

The PLA did not play a high-profile role in the 2003 SARS. Nevertheless, military forces were mobilized on a large scale in response to Covid-19. On 2 February, Xi deployed 1,400 medical staff from the armed forces to treat patients in Huoshenshan Hospital, one of the two makeshift hospitals dedicated to Covid-19 infected patients. Huoshenshan Hospital was formally delivered to military medics on 2 February [20].

On 13 February, Xi deployed 2,600 more military medics to virus-hit Wuhan. They were in charge of patients at Wuhan's Taikang Tongji Hospital (860 beds) and Hubei Provincial Women and Children's Hospital (700 beds), running services similar to their colleagues at Huoshenshan Hospital, which was already in full-scale operation [21]. The medical team consisted of personnel from units including the Ground Force, Navy, Air Force, Rocket Force, and Strategic Support Force.

More importantly, the PLA played a vital role in developing China's vaccines against Covid-19. China successfully controlled SARS in 2003 without producing any specific vaccines, while even in the early stage of the Covid-19 pandemic, a PLA research team led by military scientist Dr. Chen Wei was busy working in a makeshift lab for research and testing of Covid-19 vaccines [22]. About 50 days after the lockdown of Wuhan, the first vaccine was ready for clinical trials. In 2018, Chen was sent from China to Sierra Leone to help the African country fight against the deadly Ebola, and with a real vaccine, which showed that the PLA had accumulated experience and know-how on vaccination development even before the outbreak of Covid-19.

5. China's System of Responding to Public Emergencies

China's national system on responses to public emergencies was formalized in 2006 when the State Council enacted the National

Master Plan for Responding to Public Emergencies based on lessons learnt from the SARS outbreak in 2003. The system includes contingency plans on four categories of public emergencies, namely, public health emergencies, natural disasters, accidents, and events threatening public security. The State Council has been designated the highest administrative apparatus in charge of responses for all public emergencies [23].

The State Council has set up a four-level response system on all emergencies based on their severity and controllability, namely, Level I (most severe, red-coded), Level II (very severe, orange-coded), Level III (severe, yellow-coded), and Level IV (general, blue-coded) [23]. Any public emergency that falls into Level I or II category should be reported to the State Council within four hours after the occurrence [23].

According to the National Plan for Responding to Public Health Emergencies (国家突发公共卫生事件应急预案), which was also enacted in 2006, the government should activate Level I emergency response immediately if it is the spread of any contagious SARS-like virus or human infection from avian flu [24]. Any unidentified epidemic that involves cases in multiple provinces also deserves Level I response [24]. According to the National Master Plan for Responding to Public Emergencies, information on the occurrence of any public emergency should be publicized as soon as possible.

Under the leadership of the State Council, the National Health Commission[ii] should play a pivotal role in organising and coordinating the responses to public health emergencies [25]. The Chinese Centre for Disease Control and Prevention, a national agency under the National Health Commission, is especially important for national responses to public emergencies caused by epidemics.

[ii]The National Health Commission is a cabinet-level executive department under the State Council, which is responsible for sanitation and health in China. Throughout most of China's rule since 1949, the national health portfolio had been the responsibility of the Ministry of Health until 2013, which was superseded by the National Health and Family Planning Commission. In March 2018, the National Health and Family Planning Commission was dissolved and its functions were integrated into the new agency called the National Health Commission.

Despite the State Council's effort to set up a national system in response to public emergencies after the SARS outbreak 17 years ago, the authorities still failed to curb Covid-19 at the early stage. The contagious coronavirus is not only challenging the fulfillment of the government's ambitious economic blueprint in 2020, but also testing CCP's plan on governance capacity building. An overhaul of the national system of managing public health emergencies is very likely after the Covid-19 has been gradually brought under control.

Appendix

Timeline of Chinese Government's Reactions toward Outbreak of Covid-19 (by 24 February 2020)

31 December 2019: China alerted WHO of several cases of unusual pneumonia in Wuhan city in the central Hubei province. The virus was unknown.

3 January 2020: Dr Li Wenliang was apprehended by Wuhan local police for spreading "rumors" that a SARS-like virus was spreading in Wuhan.

5 January 2020: Chinese officials ruled out the possibility that this was a recurrence of the SARS virus.

7 January 2020: Officials announced they had identified a new virus, according to the WHO. The novel virus was named 2019-nCoV and was identified as belonging to the coronavirus family. On the same day, Xi Jinping issued demands during a Politburo Standing Committee meeting for work to contain the outbreak.

11 January 2020: China announced its first death from the virus, a 61-year-old man who had purchased goods from the seafood market.

20 January 2020: Zhong Nanshan, a Chinese expert on infectious diseases, confirmed human-to-human transmission to state

(Continued)

broadcaster CCTV, raising fears of a major outbreak on the eve of the Lunar New Year holiday. Xi gave special instructions to work on preventing and controlling the outbreak, emphasizing that the government had to pay high attention to it.

22 January 2020: The death toll in China jumped to 17, with more than 550 infections.

23 January 2020: Wuhan was placed under effective quarantine as air and rail departures were suspended. Beijing cancelled events for the Lunar New Year, while officials reported the first death outside Hubei province.

25 January 2020: Travel restrictions were imposed on a further five cities in Hubei, and 30 out of 31 provinces in China had activated the highest-level emergency response for public health (Level I).

26 January 2020: A LSG on the prevention and control of the outbreak of new pneumonia caused by the novel coronavirus was established at the central government level led by Premier Li Keqiang and with Politburo Standing Committee member Wang Huning as the deputy leader. Meanwhile another two *ad hoc* institutions were respectively set up at the central and local levels to ensure the supervision and implementation of directives from Beijing. Vice Premier Sun Chunlan headed the central government group to guide epidemic control work in Hubei province (中央赴湖北指导组), which supervised the local government's work against coronavirus, while Hubei party secretary and governor led epidemic control headquarters in Hubei province.

28 January 2020: Xi Jinping met the executive director of the WHO, Dr Tedros Adhanom Ghebreyesus and told Tedros that he "personally directed" the government's response to the outbreak.

2 February 2020: Xi deployed 1,400 medical staff from the armed forces to Huoshenshan Hospital in Wuhan city. Huoshenshan

(Continued)

(Continued)

Hospital, with a capacity of 1,000 beds, is one of the two make-shift hospitals dedicated to treating patients infected with the novel coronavirus. It was formally delivered to military medics on 2 February.

3 February 2020: In a speech to the Politburo Standing Committee, Xi outlined a contingency plan to respond to a crisis that he said could not only hamper the health of people in China, but also jeopardize the country's economic and social stability, including its Open Door Policy.

7 February 2020: Dr Li Wenliang died of Covid-19, sparking collective anger and grief on Chinese social media. The National Supervisory Commission sent an inspection group to Wuhan to thoroughly investigate issues related to Li.

10 February 2020: Xi Jinping presided over a meeting and listened to reports on epidemic prevention and control work in Beijing. Meanwhile, many enterprises in China resumed production to ensure the supply of protective materials and other products on the market to fight against the novel coronavirus epidemic.

13 February 2020: Beijing removed Hubei provincial Party Secretary Jiang Chaoliang and Wuhan municipal Party Secretary Ma Guoqiang over botched outbreak response. Shanghai Mayor Ying Yong, 61, a close ally of Xi Jinping, was named the new party boss of Hubei province, while Wang Zhonglin, 57, the party secretary of Jinan, the capital city of the eastern province of Shandong, was appointed party secretary of Wuhan city.

13 February 2020: Xi deployed 2,600 more military medics to Wuhan's Taikang Tongji Hospital (860 beds) and Hubei Provincial Women and Children's Hospital (700 beds), running services similar to their colleagues at Huoshenshan Hospital.

14 February 2020: First temporary Traditional Chinese medicines (TCM) hospital received Covid-19 patients in Wuhan.

(Continued)

19 February 2020: The National Health Commission issued an updated version of the diagnosis and treatment plan for Covid-19.

20 February 2020: In his letter to Bill Gates, co-chair of the Bill & Melinda Gates Foundation, Xi wrote: "I deeply appreciate the act of generosity of the Bill & Melinda Gates Foundation and your letter of solidarity to the Chinese people at such an important moment."

21 February 2020: Local authorities said Wuhan planned to build another 19 makeshift hospitals to receive more infected patients.

23 February 2020: The Chinese authorities released a document listing measures to strengthen protection and care for medical workers, as part of efforts to fight against the novel coronavirus outbreak.

23 February 2020: At a teleconference that was unprecedentedly open to every county government and every military regiment throughout the country, Xi Jinping said the coronavirus epidemic was the country's most serious public health crisis and promised more pro-growth policies to help overcome it.

Source: Compiled by the author.

References

[1] Human-to-human transmission confirmed in China coronavirus. https://time.com/5768404/china-coronavirus-human-transmission/, accessed 17 February 2020.

[2] Coronavirus Disease 2019 (COVID-19) situation summary. https://www.nih.gov/health-information/coronavirus, accessed 17 February 2020.

[3] Wang Huning: The low-profile, liberal dream weaver who's about to become China's ideology tsar. https://www.scmp.com/news/china/policies-politics/article/2116964/wang-huning-low-profile-liberal-dream-weaver-whos-about, accessed 17 February 2020.

[4] Where's Xi? China's leader commands Coronavirus fight from safe heights.S https://economictimes.indiatimes.com/news/international/world-news/wheres-xi-chinas-leader-commands-coronavirus-fight-from-safe-heights/articleshow/74043927.cms?from=mdr, accessed 17 February 2020.

[5] Xi urges resolute action in all-out, people's war against virus. https://www.fmprc.gov.cn/mfa_eng/zxxx_662805/t1743314.shtml , accessed 17 February 2020.

[6] State Council releases National Master Plan for Responding to Public Emergencies. http://www.gov.cn/jrzg/2006-01/08/content_150878.htm, accessed 17 February 2020.

[7] Article 1.3, China's National Plan for Responding to Public Health Emergencies (in Chinese). http://www.gov.cn/yjgl/2006-02/26/content_211654.htm, accessed 21 February 2020.

[8] Coronavirus: Beijing purges Communist Party heads in Hubei over 'botched' outbreak response in provincial capital of Wuhan. https://www.scmp.com/news/china/politics/article/3050372/coronavirus-beijings-purge-over-virus-takes-down-top-communist, accessed 18 February 2020.

[9] Ying Yong becomes Hubei Party Secretary, and Wang Zhonglin becomes Wuhan Party Secretary (in Chinese). https://m.thepaper.cn/newsDetail_forward_5964830, accessed 18 February 2020.

[10] Former Wuhan official to guide prevention and control efforts. http://www.chinadaily.com.cn/a/202002/11/WS5e41f84fa3101282172767bc.html, accessed 18 February 2020.

[11] Xi Jinping 'put China's top echelon on notice' in early days of coronavirus outbreak. *South China Morning Post*, 15 February 2020. https://www.scmp.com/news/china/politics/article/3050815/xi-jinping-put-chinas-top-echelon-notice-early-days-coronavirus accessed 18 February 2020.

[12] Chen, G. (2016). *The Politics of Disaster Management in China*, New York: Palgrave Macmillan, p. 112.

[13] Chen, G., and Xue, J. (2018). China's massive restructure of Party and State Apparatus in 2018. *EAI Background Brief*, No. 1358.

[14] Chinese vice premier inspects newly-delivered hospital to combat coronavirus. http://www.xinhuanet.com/english/2020-02/03/c_138750379.htm, accessed 19 February 2020.

[15] Taking credit, avoiding blame? Xi Jinping's absence from coronavirus frontline. https://www.theguardian.com/world/2020/feb/04/

blame-xi-jinping-absence-coronavirus-frontline-china-crisis, accessed 19 February 2020.

[16] Death of coronavirus doctor Li Wenliang becomes catalyst for 'freedom of speech' demands in China. https://www.scmp.com/news/china/politics/article/3049606/coronavirus-doctors-death-becomes-catalyst-freedom-speech, accessed 19 February 2020.

[17] Alexander, D. (2006). Globalization of disaster: Trends, problems and dilemmas. *Journal of International Affairs*, **59**(2), 11.

[18] Ross, A. D. (2014). *Local Disaster Resilience: Administrative and Political Perspectives*, New York: Routledge, p. 2.

[19] Online revolt in China as a doctor is lionized. *The New York Times*, 8 February 2020, p. 1.

[20] Xi Jinping approves sending 1,400 military medical staff to Huoshenshan Hospital in Wuhan. https://news.cgtn.com/news/2020-02-02/Military-medical-staff-to-treat-patients-in-Huoshenshan-Hospital-NKECxLtqxO/index.html, accessed 20 February 2020.

[21] Xi Jinping orders 2,600 more military medics to virus-hit Wuhan. https://news.cgtn.com/news/2020-02-13/Xi-approves-sending-2-600-military-medical-workers-to-Wuhan--O2JiE4f1Ty/index.html, accessed 20 February 2020.

[22] Chen Wei: She-power behind China's first COVID-19 vaccine. *CGTN News*, 8 September 2020, https://news.cgtn.com/news/2020-09-08/Chen-Wei-She-power-behind-China-s-first-COVID-19-vaccine-TBboFN0Qbm/index.html, accessed 15 April 2021.

[23] Interpreting National Master Plan for Responding to Public Emergencies (in Chinese). http://www.gov.cn/zwhd/2006-01/08/content_151018.htm, accessed 21 February 2020.

[24] Article 1.3, China's National Plan for Responding to Public Health Emergencies (in Chinese). http://www.gov.cn/yjgl/2006-02/26/content_211654.htm, accessed 21 February 2020.

[25] Article 2.1, China's National Plan for Responding to Public Health Emergencies (in Chinese). http://www.gov.cn/yjgl/2006-02/26/content_211654.htm, accessed 21 February 2020.

https://doi.org/10.1142/9789811255151_0007

Chapter 7

ASEAN–China Relations in New Normal with Covid-19

Linda Low

Singapore University of Social Sciences, Singapore

1. Introduction

This chapter discusses how the Association of Southeast Asian Nations (ASEAN10), as a group, features in the Covid-19 period. ASEAN was founded with five members, Indonesia, Malaysia, Singapore, Thailand, and the Philippines, and has grown to 10 members at present after Cambodia, Laos, Myanmar, and Vietnam (CLMV) and Brunei joined to form ASEAN10 (Figure 1).

On 31 July 1961, when ASEAN was mooted and formed, it was then called the Association of Southeast Asia (ASA), as a group comprising Thailand, the Philippines, and the Federation of Malaya. On 8 August 1967, the foreign ministers of five countries: Indonesia, Malaysia, the Philippines, Singapore, and Thailand, signed the ASEAN Declaration, paving way for the formation of ASEAN. As set out in the ASEAN Declaration, the aims and purposes of ASEAN are to accelerate economic growth, social progress, and cultural development, among other areas.

From the beginning, ASEAN chose to be in the Non-Aligned Movement (NAM). However, historically, the US was the main

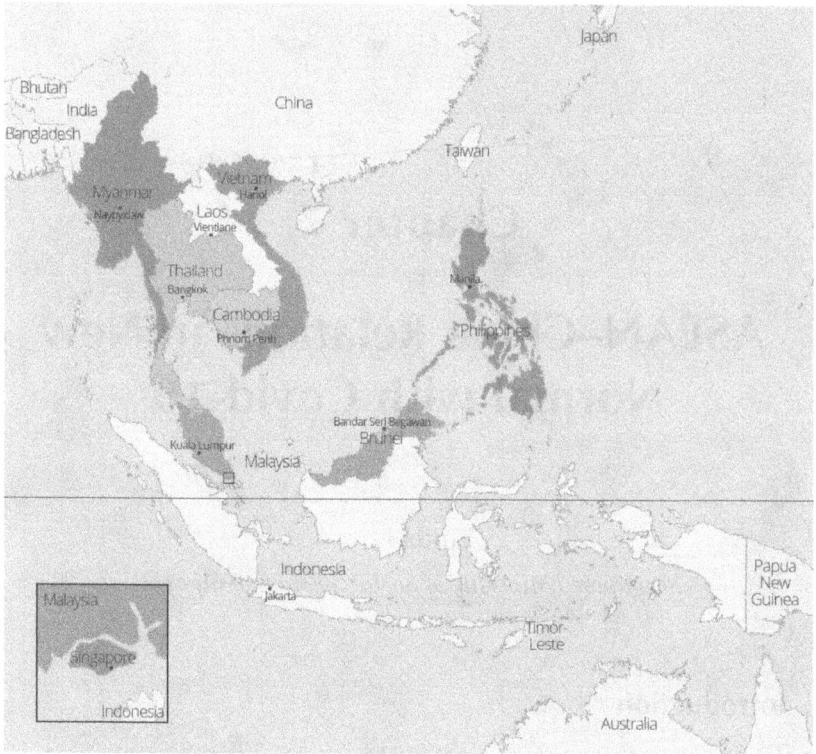

Figure 1. ASEAN10 members.

influential nation in the ASEAN region, with the Philippines being its former main colony and the UK having colonial history in Malaysia, Singapore and Brunei. Interestingly, Thailand, standing literally as free land, was never colonized. Although ASEAN follows NAM in theory, a rising China that poses a challenge to the US in the main aspects of geopolitics and geoeconomics, as it began opening up to trade and investment among other areas, presented certain dilemmas to ASEAN10 as a group. This is not surprising as the US and China are generally seen as geopolitical rivals.

Lee Kuan Yew foresaw this prospect, and slanted toward China as he chose for Singapore as mainly Chinese in racial composition. Thus, Singapore follows mainland China's Hanyu-pinyin rather than traditional Mandarin followed in the territories of Hong Kong and Taiwan. Rightly or not, Lee opted to build closer ties with China in trade and, with China being the most populous country in the world, in all socio-economic matters.

Historically, ASEAN was vital to the West, especially for the US and Europe, and remains as important to China in purely economic terms, as a food basket and source of natural resources — from rubber and tin in Malaysia to Thai rice — among other such resources that are richly-abundant in ASEAN-rich economies.

In political matters, while ASEAN in theory follows NAM, in practice it leans closer to China than the US, which is also withdrawing somewhat from the Asia-Pacific region to focus on its immediate neighborhood, such as Canada, Mexico, and other countries. In that sense, ASEAN is caught up in Sino–US rivalry in geoeconomic and geopolitical matters. It is simply a practical choice, as in the case of the then Filipino President Rodrigo Duterte, who visited Xi Jinping in Beijing many times since assuming office in 2016. His fifth visit in three years was from 28 August to 1 September 2019. That he had not made a single trip to the US in his presidential capacity is rather telling.

Historically, while the Philippines was a former US colony and long-time ally of the US, since Duterte took office in 2016, Filipino–Sino ties have been warming up. Among other matters, the Filipino affinity to China clearly also affects ASEAN NAM standing. China need not consciously woo ASEAN, thereby affecting ASEAN NAM, as seen in Lee Kuan Yew's choice in the adoption of China's Hanyu Pinyin for Singapore. Singapore may even rival Hong Kong in Chinese trade and investment, as Hong Kong grapples with their relationship to mainland China for its own geopolitical reasons, if not geoeconomics, as Shanghai among other Chinese cities grew in significance as well to rival Hong Kong.

On the other hand, the Filipino public were critical of President Rodrigo Duterte's Beijing-friendly stance. Perhaps like Singapore's choice of China's Hanyu-pinyin, the Philippines aims to strengthen economic rather than political ties in theoretical terms to forge a stronger relationship with China. How Singapore may show the practical side of its Chinese relationship as also affecting ASEAN is perhaps not its main reasoning. For the Singapore city-state, it is pure practical survival. Oddly, Hong Kong as more political-minded may do well for Singapore city-state.

As long as China is not seen or perceived as interfering or consciously dividing ASEAN NAM to divert ASEAN to adopt a Sino-friendly rather than a traditionally US stand, geoeconomics prove practical. In theory, ASEAN can continue to follow NAM. In practice, Sino–ASEAN trade and foreign direct investment (FDI) are clearly significant, with the US also withdrawing somewhat from Southeast Asia and the ASEAN region, especially since the Vietnam War, among other geopolitical and geoeconomic matters. Was Duterte proving to be practical in going the Sino way? Or is it possible that China has not realized Duterte's intentions for his pro-China stand?

In theory, Singapore remains neutral in accordance with NAM, but in practice it has chosen China's Hanyu-pinyin as its second language after English for practical rather than historical reasons as a former British colony. In contrast, the territories of Hong Kong and Taiwan use traditional Mandarin, not Hanyu-pinyin. In some instances, Singapore has to be practical rather than be historically and politically inclined as China rises to be a vital economic force in trade and investment. In any case, Chinese communist ideology poses little to no threat to Singapore today. Therefore, as Hong Kong chooses to be less Sino-inclined, is Singapore stepping right up?

2. China in Singapore's Context

The above is clear when one looks at where and how Singapore stands, both as an ASEAN member and as an independent sovereign city-state. While Hong Kong is naturally closer geographically and economically as China's trade and investment hub, Hong Kong's politics are not as clear-cut for good reasons, and thereby not as friendly as that of Sino–Singapore. In many senses and ways, a good, practical economic relationship between China and Singapore proves to be beneficial to the rest of ASEAN as well.

3. China in Regional Context

As noted, ASEAN is an important, if not main, source for food and natural resources to help China sustain its position as the Factory-of-the-World and Consumer-of-the-World. Singapore serves as an intermediate port and airport among others, cementing the city-state's relevance to China. The combined ASEAN population is about half of that of China, which also provides a significant weight-age to the Sino–ASEAN relationship.

In practical geopolitics, ASEAN, including Singapore, would rather have less competition and conflict between China and the West, the US in particular. How NAM works out is as clear as mud again; Singapore in practice is China-oriented while not posing as any conscious rival or threat to Hong Kong as China's entrepot. Strangely, Singapore, as an independent sovereign state, is unlike Hong Kong, which was neither independent as an ex-British colony nor is affiliated to China in that political sense. Oddly and strangely, China as the Factory-of-the-World and Consumer-of-the-World, also emerged as the epicenter of Covid-19, first discovered in Wuhan.

On another front in defense, in 2017, Malaysia–China's defense relationship peaked after former Prime Minister Najib Razak renewed the Memorandum of Understanding (MoU) on defense cooperation during his trip to Beijing in October 2016. The visit came months after a special arbitral tribunal ruled in favor of the Philippines in its dispute with Beijing over its South China Sea claims. The Najib government seemed determined not let that landmark case affect its pursuit of closer ties with China. Its efforts appeared to pay off, with many top-level exchanges, large-scale bilateral exercises, continued military academic exchanges, and even two submarine visits taking place. Sensitive visits to Sepanggar naval base in Kota Kinabalu took place despite Malaysia being a claimant of the contested waterway.

About 5 years on, Malaysia's defense establishment has become increasing skeptical of China–Malaysia defense ties. That slowed in part due to changes in government, political instability, and no less, the coronavirus pandemic. A classic case of success in economics turning to political ambitions is classically geoeconomics turning into geopolitics.

China's more assertive stance in the South China Sea is clear in Spratly Islands, Diaoyu, and Bay of Bengal — are they all signs that a storm is brewing in the Asia-Pacific waters? A start to cooling bilateral relations began in May 2018 as Mahathir Mohamad's coalition removed previous administration's 6-decade grip on power in the general election. Under Najib's leadership, there were high-level defense exchanges, including a 2016 visit by China's People's Liberation Army (PLA) Chief of Staff Fang Fenghui to officiate the bilateral Aman Youyi military exercise.

In March 2017, Vice-Chairman Central Military Commission Xu Qiliang, who ranks higher than China's defense minister, became the highest-ranked PLA officer to visit Malaysia and met both Najib and defense minister Hishammuddin Hussein to deepen consensus and widen areas of defense cooperation. However, bilateral visits fell sharply after Mahathir became the Prime Minister, although Malaysian officials did attend the Xiangshan Forum, a regional security dialogue that China first established in 2006, with a ceremony to receive the first littoral mission ship (LMS). Interest in Chinese weaponry remained among the Malaysian political leadership, given its competitive prices, although it was somewhat less favored by the professional military, which viewed China-made weapons as solid, but not spectacular.

The LMS is part of Malaysian navy's modernization program to reduce current 15 classes of vessels to five. A total of 18 LMS were to be procured under this plan, with the China Shipbuilding Industry Corporation bagging the contract to build the first four. The original 1.17 billion ringgit (US$285 million) agreement was signed in 2017 to construct two vessels in China, with the other two in Malaysia, so Malaysia's Boustead Naval Shipyard could benefit from the technology-skill transfers, but in March 2019, Mahathir's officials renegotiated the deal so all four ships were built in the Chinese shipyard, at a slightly reduced cost of 1.047b ringgit (US$255 million).

In October 2020, *Janes*, the defense news magazine, reported deficiencies in the first LMS, KD Keris, mainly involving sensors and combat systems, and it was reported that the Chinese contractors were asked to improve the remaining hulls. Ironically, KD Keris was deployed by the navy in November 2020 to monitor China Coast Guard vessel in Luconia Shoals, where the stand-off is believed to have occurred. Malaysia decided to seek other foreign partners to build the remaining LMSs. Now another major procurement from China remains unlikely, although China-made weapon systems remain in contention in some procurement programs. For example, the JF-17 fighter, jointly produced by China and Pakistan, and the L-15B lead-in fighter-trainer, developed by China's Hongdu, are both contenders for Malaysia's light aviation combat aircraft project. Following the political coup in February 2020, Malaysia had another change in government, which coincided with its rapidly growing challenge to combat Covid-19.

Understandably, activities related to defense diplomacy were scaled down due to Covid-19, however, an exception was the September 2020 visit by China's Minister of Defense Wei Fenghe. He met then Prime Minister Muhyiddin Yassin and then Defense Minister Ismail Sabri Yaakob. They discussed South China Sea, cooperation in the pandemic, and strengthening defense cooperation, among other issues.

On paper, the Muhyiddin government appointed two veterans of the Najib cabinet to helm defense and foreign ministries — in particular, the appointment of Hishammuddin as Foreign Minister should be advantageous to rekindle Malaysia–China defense ties versus an inherently unstable government that was consumed and distracted by constant domestic politicking and pandemic and which did not consider defense diplomacy with China as a high priority.

Chinese actions in the South China Sea also contribute to reduced enthusiasm, increased skepticism by defense establishment, and less efficacy to develop defense relations with China. The West Capella episode in April 2020, in which a Chinese government survey ship tagged an exploration vessel operated by the Malaysian state oil company Petronas in the South China Sea was especially alarming to the establishment. While bilateral defense interactions are still valued as a channel of trust and confidence building, they are now met with more skepticism compared to the early 2010s.

Yet, Duterte was to visit China to thank Xi for its Covid-19 vaccine donation as reported on February 28, 2021. In contrast to the traditional ASEAN–US relationships, China is clearly stepping up as the US gradually withdraws from the Asia-Pacific region. One may even question whether ASEAN's continuing allegiance to NAM, at least on paper, is still relevant as definitely the region is more Sino-inclined now. ASEAN's regional role amid the Myanmar crisis and China–US tensions are evident. The Myanmar coup opened up a new front of debate on ASEAN and its ability to response to urgent regional crises. Such questions are not new. The perennial challenge posed by South China Sea disputes and the deeper issue of growing China–US rivalry make some critics wonder whether ASEAN can still function as meaningfully as an institution, or whether the days of ASEAN centrality are numbered?

For instance, studies were conducted by the Centre for Non-Traditional Security Studies (NTS Centre) at the S. Rajaratnam School of International Studies (RSIS), in Nanyang Technological University (NTU) in Singapore. Be it Covid-19 or issues of politics or economics, all have to reckon with China as the power. Strategic resilience in Southeast Asia and ASEAN has been touted as a break from the past toward a better prepared post-pandemic future in the region. The term focuses on strategic supply chain resilience. However, within the regional context of a people-centered ASEAN, a more comprehensive understanding of strategic resilience is needed to move beyond a narrow focus on supply chains. Without a recalibration of the term, it may signal a snap back to a pre-Covid era or "old" ways of thinking. The term captures the mutually reinforcing nature of strategic thinking and resilience. It is therefore timely to redress this imbalance to use strategic thinking to inform a more sustainable and resilient future in Southeast Asia and ASEAN.

All these issues pose a challenge to cooperation within a fragmented global system. Regional cooperation within a fragmented global system has faced significant challenges in responding to the Covid-19 pandemic, from disruption of supply chains and movement of people, disproportionate effects on marginalized communities, and poor pandemic preparedness and planning to emergence of vaccine nationalism. As the Covid-19 pandemic continues to evolve, regional cooperation, particularly in Asia, has reemerged as an important component to secure vaccines, recalibrate supply chains, negotiate travel lanes, and share knowledge of public health safety practices for benefit of the region and its people.

Given the successes achieved so far under crisis conditions, it is important to utilize this experience to move decision-makers' mind-sets away from reactive measures toward investing in a longer-term vision to engage people and build sustainable and strategic resilience for the future. So, what does it all mean? The key elements for ASEAN is: to develop a more holistic understanding of strategic resilience aims to inform states, companies, and societies at large on how to recover quickly in times of disruption and become future-ready. It does so by securing four key elements: evidence-based decision-making, institutional capability, organizational leadership, and societal adaptability. All are reliant on the capability to ensure strong organizations, systems, and human resources through learning, development, skills, and experience. In ASEAN, there are key operational institutions developed within sectors with implications for wider ASEAN security governance, from the well-established ASEAN Coordinating Centre on Humanitarian Assistance in disaster management to more direct relevant institutions.

An announcement of a feasibility study on an ASEAN Centre on Public Health Emergencies and Emerging Diseases is relevant. These could form an implementation arm of regional cooperation, such as the ASEAN Agreement on Disaster Management and Emergency Response. The need to synergize actions is clear; however, implementation is always the hardest part in regional cooperation. Clearly, linkages across sectors are limited, so there is need to synergize their actions with broader strategic resilience within the regional community. This would build a more robust system that would inform contingency planning for future pandemics and other potential challenging scenarios. In the year 2020, it became acutely apparent that not only does regional cooperation matter but also, importantly, it should include engagement with extra-regional actors, particularly those producing vaccines. It underlines interconnections between countries in Southeast Asia and the wider world.

The Covid-19 pandemic further caused restrictions on movement of people both within and outside countries of residence. Restrictions have a disproportionate effect on marginalized communities within countries of residence, and it has curtailed the global movement of people. As countries gradually open up, beginning with travel bubbles between those with effective pandemic response, it further underlines the importance of investment in effective governance systems. As countries in the region move forward, there should be a greater focus on whole-of-society approaches to tackle pandemic and its disproportionate impacts — such as through the implementation of ASEAN Comprehensive Recovery Framework — and it is important to consider potential future crises to develop vision to achieve strategic resilience in region.

4. Conclusion

Figures 2 to 7 serve as a pictorial conclusion to further spark ideas.

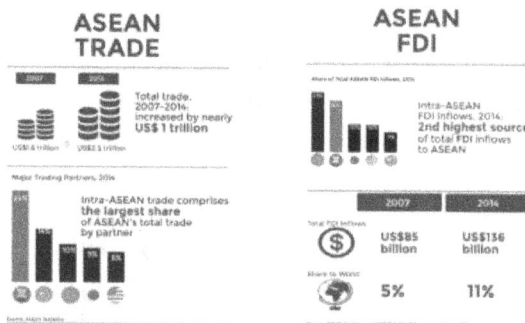

Figure 2.   Open economies: Trade and FDI.

Source: Adapted from https://twitter.com/analyseasia/status/691447937998675970/photo/1.

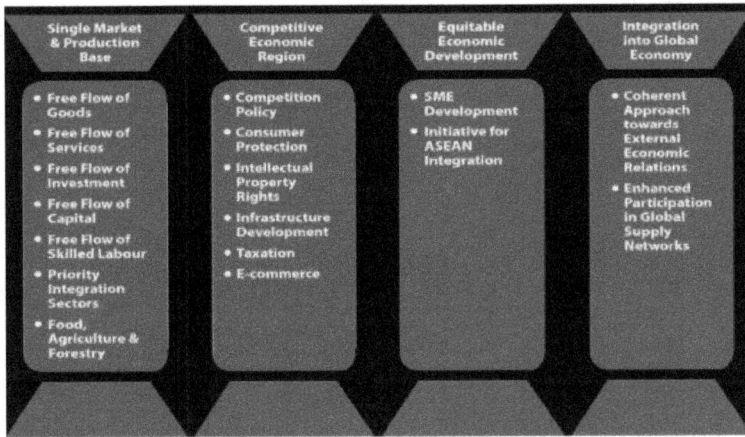

Figure 3. ASEAN Economic Community 2015.

Source: Adapted from http://asean.dla.go.th/public/article.do?lv2Index=83&lang=en&ran
dom=1474735020852.

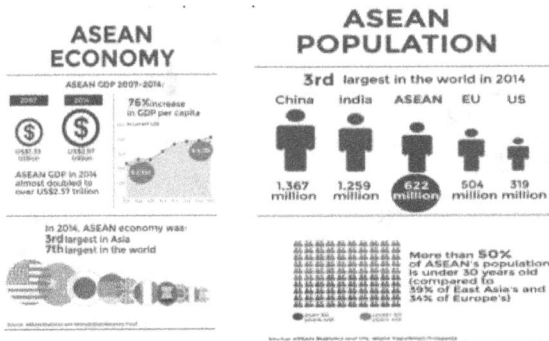

Figure 4. ASEAN GDP US$2.5 trillion. The average GDP per capita grew 80% to US$4,000, 2007–2014.

Source: Adapted from https://www.weforum.org/agenda/2017/01/asean-is-50-and-it-s-come-a-long-way-here-s-why-you-should-care/.

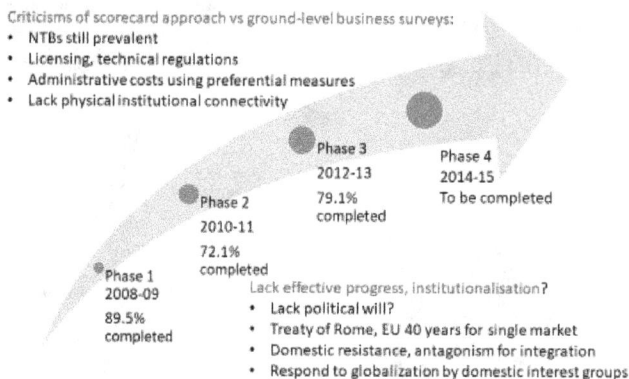

Criticisms of scorecard approach vs ground-level business surveys:
- NTBs still prevalent
- Licensing, technical regulations
- Administrative costs using preferential measures
- Lack physical institutional connectivity

Phase 3
2012-13
79.1%
completed

Phase 4
2014-15
To be completed

Phase 2
2010-11
72.1%
completed

Phase 1
2008-09
89.5%
completed

Lack effective progress, institutionalisation?
- Lack political will?
- Treaty of Rome, EU 40 years for single market
- Domestic resistance, antagonism for integration
- Respond to globalization by domestic interest groups

Figure 5. ASEAN Economic Community blueprint: 2008–2013 as 77.54% completed.

Source: Adapted from https://asean.org/asean-economic-community/.

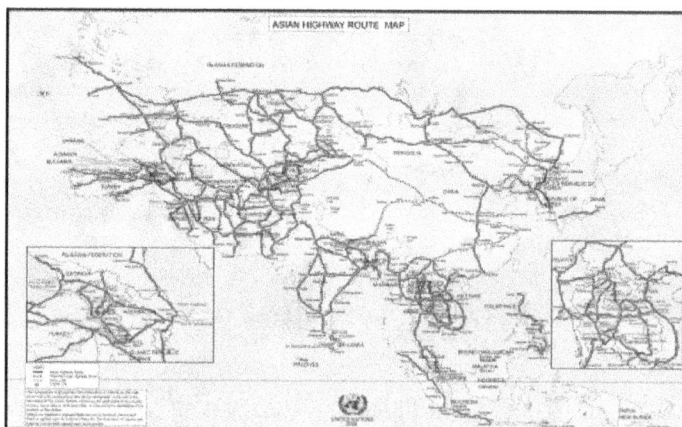

Figure 6. Suggested potential trans-Asian highway route by United Nations: Is ASEAN the stepping stone?

Source: Adapted from https://www.unescap.org/sites/default/files/Full%20version.pdf.

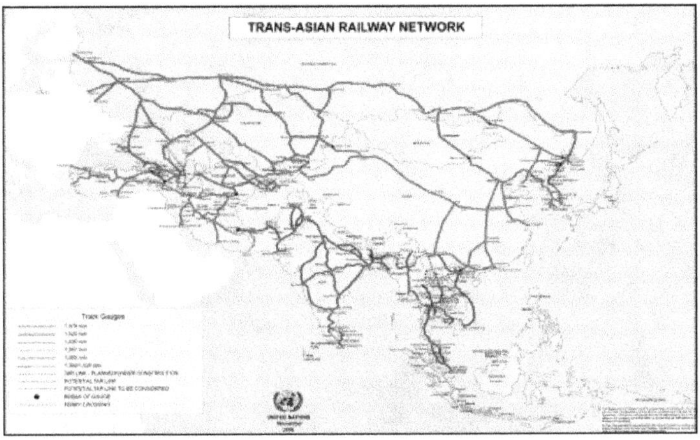

Figure 7. Suggested potential trans-Asian railway route by United Nations: Is ASEAN the stepping stone?

Source: Adapted from https://www.unescap.org/sites/default/files/Lao%20PDR%20country%20report-TAR%20WGM-5.pdf.

Chapter 8

Covid-19 in Southeast Asia: A Review of the Current Scenario and Outlook for the Future

Mohan Ravuru*, Yong Poovorawan[†],
Carmenchu Echiverri-Villavicencio[‡],
Rontgene M. Solante[§], and Aw Tar Choon[¶,‖]

*Abbott Rapid Diagnostics, Singapore
[†]Center of Excellence in Clinical Virology Department of Pediatrics
Faculty of Medicine, Chulalongkorn University, Thailand
[‡]Department of Infectious Disease, St. Luke's Medical Center
Department of Medicine, Section of Infectious Disease
St. Luke's Global City, The Philippines
[§]Philippine College of Physicians
Philippine Society for Microbiology and Infectious Diseases
Infectious Diseases Society of America (IDSA)
San Lazaro Hospital, Quiricada Street, Santa Cruz,
Manila, Philippines
[¶]Duke-NUS Graduate Medical School, Singapore
Changi General Hospital, Singapore

[‖]Corresponding author.

Southeast Asia (SEA), home to 675 million people, earned global appreciation for its successful containment of coronavirus disease 2019 (Covid-19) in 2020, with imposition of extensive lockdowns, travel and mobility restrictions, and ban on mass events and shutting down of businesses, factories, entertainment, and schools. The socioeconomic consequences of prolonged lockdowns and the public demand to lift mobility restrictions for annual festivals put an enormous strain on SEA countries, prompting governments to exit lockdowns without an adaptive public health strategy and preparedness. Case numbers and deaths have surged in Indonesia, the Philippines, Thailand, Malaysia, and Vietnam since April 2021, overwhelming fragile healthcare systems and exposing public health vulnerabilities. Lack of testing capacity, the rapid spread of more transmissible virus variants, and slow vaccine rollout have turned the region into an epicenter of Covid-19, with recurrent waves of infection. Scaled-up testing, accelerated vaccination, strengthening the healthcare system capacity, and appropriate use of therapeutics are imperative for securing human security, economic recovery, and political confidence. The SEA countries must respond decisively, innovatively, and together to suppress the spread of the virus and address the socioeconomic devastation that Covid-19 is causing in the region. In the long term, regional pandemic preparedness will remain essential, even as individual countries' capabilities continue to vary considerably.

1. Background

Covid-19 has entered its third calendar year, with the first cases reported toward the end of 2019. SEA was the first region to be affected outside China. Fearing the rapid spread of the pandemic, countries in the region took unprecedented measures to protect their communities. Overall, the region has done remarkably well in bringing the primary wave under control. The relative success of early lockdowns to save lives and minimize long-term economic impact seems to have culminated in a more serious secondary wave of infections in 2021 in some countries. The proportionate increases in new cases and deaths are indicative of the rise of a more severe stage of the region's Covid-19 crisis.

The surge in cases typically follows the easing of restrictions to alleviate the burden on businesses, factories, restaurants, entertainment, and social life. It is all coming at a time when economies and households are weakened by the consequences of more than a year of social restrictions, and governments are not eager to repeat the 2020 lockdowns. In essence, flattening the epidemic curve has flattened the economy and steepened the recession curve further (Figure 1).

The healthcare systems in the region have varying critical care capacities, with over 10 beds per 100,000 population in Brunei, Singapore, and Thailand but fewer than three in Indonesia, Laos, Myanmar, and the Philippines [1]. The public health consequences of the return to economic activity without a well-thought-out "exit strategy" are increasingly obvious. The current trend indicates there can be no lasting end to the economic crisis without an end to the health crisis. Several other factors contributing to the complexity of this developing crisis include inadequate testing capacity, low Covid-19 vaccination rate, and the rapid spread of severe acute respiratory syndrome coronavirus 2 (SARS-CoV-2) variants. The porous land

Evolution of the COVID-19 pandemic and the new normal

The amplitude and frequency of the subsequent waves will depend upon testing, prevention of transmission, keeping variants in check and speed of vaccination roll-out

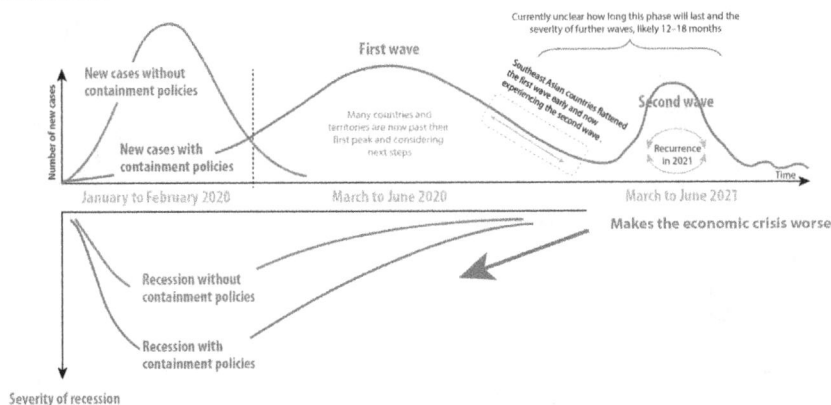

Figure 1. Impact of containment policies on epidemiological curve vs. severity of recession.

borders, large populations dispersed across diverse geographies, migrant labor force, and illegal immigration have all contributed to the ongoing humanitarian crisis.

This narrative and analytical review follows a panel discussion involving thought leaders from Thailand, the Philippines, and Singapore held in May 2021. The goal of this chapter is to review the epidemiology, review the state of the science related to Covid-19, identify challenges, and discuss the path forward for public health and economy, as SEA rounds a corner in the fight against Covid-19.

2. Epidemiology and Burden of Covid-19 in the SEA Region

SEA, with a population of more than 675 million people, has turned into a hotspot and is fast becoming the region hardest hit by recurrent waves of Covid-19, with the rate of infections and deaths racing ahead of previously worst-affected places like Latin America and India [2]. The average number of confirmed daily new cases in the region had increased from more than 12,900 in March 2021 to 28,800 in June 2021, with a median time-varying reproduction number of 1.09, which indicates that the daily new cases were growing exponentially (Figure 2) [3]. Reproduction numbers from SEA,

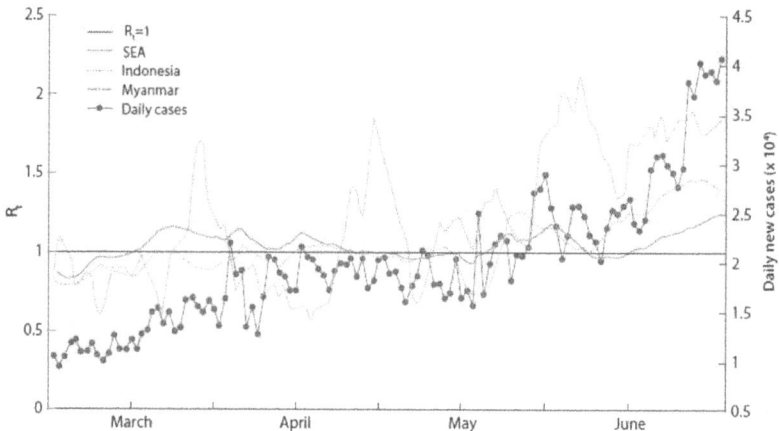

Figure 2.   An overview of COVID-19 epidemiology in Southeast Asia (as of 30 June 2021).

Indonesia (the country with the highest case number), and Myanmar are on the rise [3]. Based on existing data from Myanmar, the reproduction number has already exceeded 1.0 (Figure 2) [3].

The region had seen cases jump by around 37% between July and August 2021 to nearly 100,000 daily cases as compared to the preceding months (Figure 3A). The highest number of confirmed Covid-19 cases and consequent deaths (Figure 3B) were reported in Indonesia, the Philippines, Malaysia, Thailand, and Myanmar.

In Thailand, Indonesia, and the Philippines, hospital beds are quickly filling up after infections, overwhelming the already fragile healthcare system capacity. In Thailand, the numbers spiked after Songkran, the Thai New Year. Since then, the caseload has crept upward and has more than quadrupled to nearly 135,000 as the authorities struggled to contain outbreaks in overcrowded prisons, markets, and camps housing construction workers [4].

Overall, Covid-19 deaths reported across SEA showed an increasing trend in Indonesia, Malaysia, and the Philippines. The region has seen the highest deaths globally, as soaring infections push fragile healthcare systems to the brink and expose sluggish vaccination rollouts. The overall prevalence in the region is likely even worse than the data suggest due to the low testing capacity in many of the countries. Epidemiological models predict that the region could have as many as 2.3 million infections and 4,500 deaths each day, with more than half of all infections and deaths from Indonesia. The situation looks likely to deteriorate further, where at their peak, these countries could see as many as 75,000 daily new cases between them [5].

2.1 *Testing*

Testing and case identification are key strategies in controlling the Covid-19 pandemic. Contact tracing and isolation are only possible if cases have been identified. The frequency and percentage of tests conducted by each country are important to understand the scale of the pandemic and its impact on each country [6]. The approach of SEA has generally been to use several metrics related to testing, such as case count, test positivity rate, number of hospitalizations, and

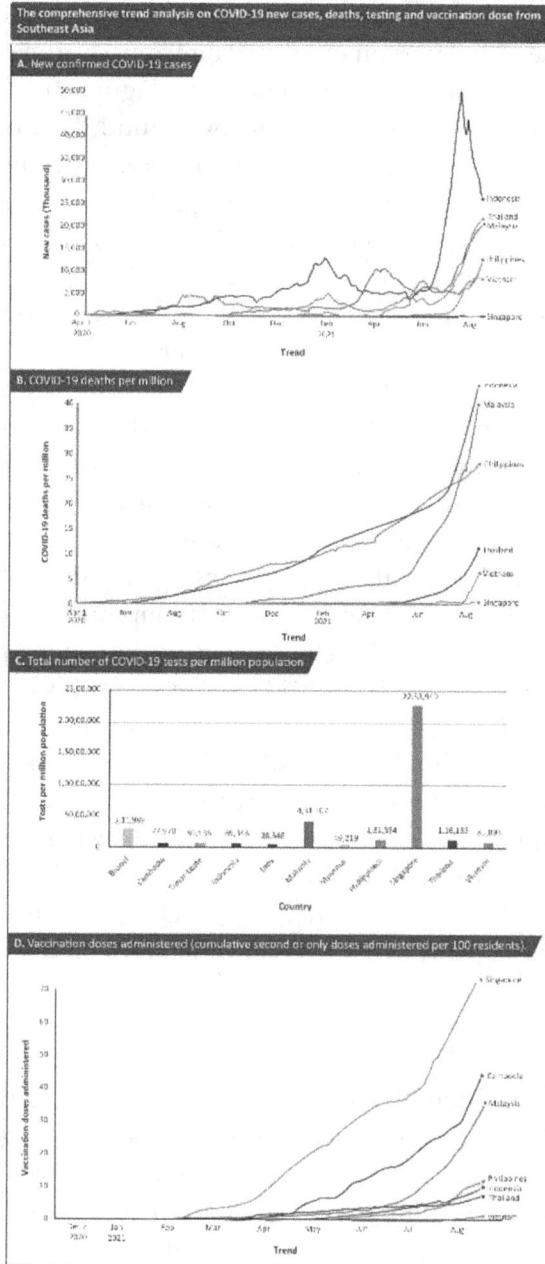

Figure 3. The comparehensive trend of COVID-19 pandemic (new cases, deaths, testing and vaccination dose) in Southeast Asia.

mortality rate, with benchmarks for each criterion that is used to justify removing or reinstating containment and mitigation measures in phases. However, many of these metrics rely on cases that have been identified through active testing of symptomatic individuals. The challenge is the substantial proportion of the infectious population that is asymptomatic, who keep the community transmission unchecked [7]. Consequently, diagnostic testing has been inadequate to reveal what proportion of the population is infected and infectious, with real infections in most countries estimated to be 10 to 15 times, and sometimes even 100 times, higher than the reported cases [8].

While the overall testing capacity in the region is low compared to the magnitude of the pandemic, Singapore performed the most number of Covid-19 tests per million population (Figure 3C). As of 20 July 2021, approximately 15.2 million Covid-19 tests had been carried out. Mass testing has been one of the ways that Singapore has managed to keep the Covid-19 pandemic under control. Testing for new Covid-19 cases has become a regular aspect of life, and mechanisms to adapt and meet this heightened demand are in place. Since the outbreak of the pandemic in early 2020, the city-state has ramped up its testing capacity from a few thousand tests per day to 60,000–70,000 tests per day [9].

2.2 *Covid-19 vaccination*

As of third quarter of 2021, the proportion of fully vaccinated population in Indonesia, the Philippines, Thailand, and Malaysia was 5%, 2.5%, 4% and 7.2%, respectively; with the highest in Singapore (42%) (Figure 3D), and vaccination rates in other SEA countries as a percentage of their population are low and slow to be implemented.

Factors affecting vaccination programs vary considerably across the SEA region but include the following [10]:

• Shortage of vaccine supply
• Limited vaccine production capabilities in the region

- Vaccine hesitancy, with reasons ranging from religious concerns that vaccines might not be halal to doubts about the efficacy and safety of vaccines. In the Philippines, the troubled introduction of a Dengue vaccination in 2016 still reverberates.
- Complex "last-mile" delivery due to difficult terrains, spread of islands, and/or dispersed populations
- Public health systems are grossly under-resourced, particularly in the lower- and middle-income countries
- Bureaucratic constraints
- Political conflicts, such as in the case of Myanmar following the military coup

3. Biology of the Virus and Transmission Dynamics

The rate of transmission of Covid-19 in the course of a pandemic is typically cyclical and wavy due to government interventions, behavioral changes, and environmental and social factors [11]. The number of infected individuals is wave-like, due to alternating periods of high and low rates of transmission. Low testing rates in the most populous SEA countries — such as Indonesia and the Philippines — are likely disguising the full extent of outbreaks, while Myanmar has seen a collapse in testing since the February 2021 coup. The true number of infections is likely to be several-fold higher than the number of confirmed cases [12].

The basic reproduction number for SARS-CoV-2 is estimated between 2 and 3. Based on that, initial estimates put the herd immunity threshold around 60%–70% to stop transmission. As the SARS-CoV-2 virus mutates and the variants dominate, the R0 changes. The proportion of population immunity correlates with the amplitude of the wave of infection: the higher the immunity, the lower the height of the wave (Figure 4) [13].

As the variants become dominant, they delay population immunity. While many people are acquiring natural immunity through infection, the proportion of people who need to be simultaneously immune also increases to achieve population immunity by 10%–20%

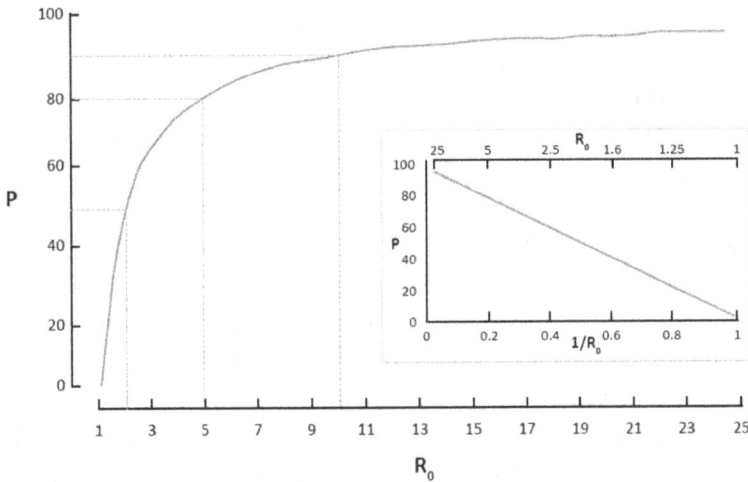

Figure 4. The relation between the basic reproduction number of a virus, R_0, and the proportion of the population that needs to be immunized to achieve immunity.

and to increase vaccine coverage levels needed to 65%–80% of the population (or 78%–95% of those over 12 years old) [14].

3.1 SARS-CoV-2 evolution and emerging variants

The SARS-CoV-2 virus has demonstrated that it can alter its genetic structures, leading to substantial changes in fundamental character-istics, including replication rate, transmission efficiency, and pathogenesis. The outbreak has seen multiple waves of infection, corresponding to the genetic variants of the virus, each with differ-ing potential public health concerns [15].

Concerns about variants are as follows:

- Mutations in the "body" of the virus (the viral genes that are expressed in infected cells and control replication and cell response) affect virus fitness and disease severity [15].
- Mutations in the spike glycoprotein affect virus transmission and antibody escape [15].

- Both vaccination and transmission rates can create positive selection pressure on the emergence and establishment of resistant strains [11].
- Recombination of the more aggressive variants could result in an even more lethal strain [16].

Covid-19 variants have been demonstrated to be associated with significant changes, such as an increase in transmissibility or detrimental change in Covid-19 epidemiology (Table 1); increase in virulence or change in clinical disease presentation; or decrease in the effectiveness of public health and social measures or available diagnostics, vaccines and therapeutics [11]. The evolution of the virus has been so rapid that the most recent Delta variant, which is currently dominating the world (Figure 5), is at least twice as transmissible as the wild-type SARS-CoV-2 virus and 60% more transmissible than its predecessor alpha variant (Table 2) [17].

According to the World Health Organization, the Delta variant is reported in 100+ countries and will continue to spread in other parts. Evidence is linked to a resurgence of Covid-19 cases and deaths in SEA [3].

Spikes in Covid-19 cases happen after the emergence of new variants, suggesting that previous infections did not confer broad enough protection to the virus. Vaccinating quickly and thoroughly can prevent a new variant, but the unevenness of vaccine rollouts and inadequate testing present a real challenge that could create evolutionary pressure to create new variants. Emerging variants have made difficult and have prolonged the development of population immunity threshold [11].

4. Current State of the Science

4.1 *Covid-19 immunity*

Covid-19 immunity is dependent upon several factors, such as age, early immune response to infection, the severity of disease, initial efficacy of a vaccine, viral variants, and comorbid health conditions [18]. We are still unsure of how long natural immunity lasts. Based

Table 1. Variants of concern and impact on transmission, reproduction number, and vaccine efficacy (as of 30 June 2021).

Variant of Concern (VOC)	First Identified	# Countries Reporting	Transmissibility vs Original Strain	Reproduction Number (RO)	Impact on Vaccine Efficacy*
α Alpha B.1.1.7	United Kingdom, September 2020	118	59%–74% increase	3.75	Minimal reduction
β Beta B.1.351	South Africa, May 2020	64	~50% increase	3.75	Minimal reduction
γ Gamma P.1	Brazil, November 2020	38	N/A	N/A	Significant reduction
δ Delta B.1.617.2	India, October 2020	>100	110–180% increase	5–8	Significant reduction

*as measured by neutralization by convalescent and post-vaccination sera

Variants of interest	
ε Epsilon	B1427/B1429, 5 March 2021, United States
ζ Zeta	P2, 17 March 2021, Brazil
η Eta	B1525, 17 March 2021, Multiple countries
Θ Theta	P3, 24 March 2021, The Philippines
ι Iota	B1526, 24 March 2021, United States
κ Kappa	B16171, 4 April 2021, India

Source: WHO, GISAID, LSHTM reports.

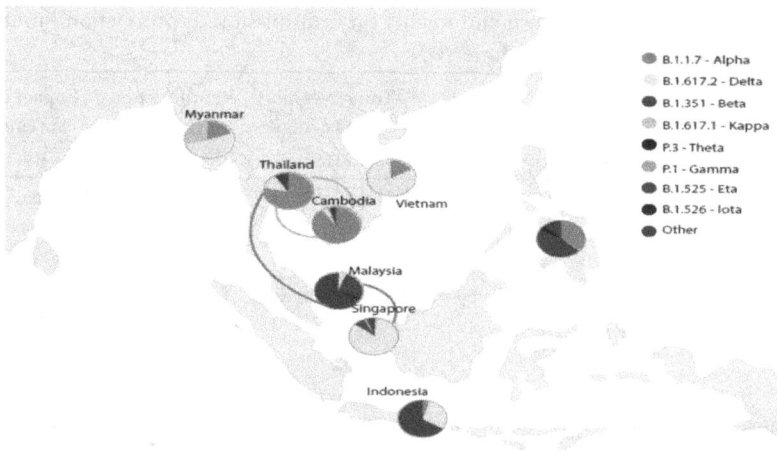

Figure 5. SARS-CoV-2 variant distribution in Southeast Asia.

Table 2. Comparison of antibody response to natural infection.

Group	Antibody Status	% of Patients	Projected Days to 50% Protection
Negative	Detectable levels never reached	11.6	—
Rapid waning	Detectable levels in 20 days but decline in <180 days	29.8	90
Slow waning	Detectable 180 days post-infection	29	125
Persistent	Negligible decay for many months	31.7	>1 year
Delayed response	Late surge of levels post-recovery	1.8	>1 year

on other severe coronavirus infections, immunity probably lasts months to years, but it is not lifelong. Immunity may also be less protective in patients who have had a mild or asymptomatic disease. If immunity is not long-lasting, or if people with a mild infection do not develop immunity, population immunity cannot be achieved without a vaccine. Covid-19 also has much higher rates of severe illness than many other viral infections, with up to 15% of infected people being hospitalized and mortality rates estimated at 0.5% to 1%. These rates are several times higher than seasonal influenza [18].

4.2 *Natural acquired immunity*

Researchers in Singapore found that Covid-19 patients and the antibody levels following the infection fall into five groups (Table 2). The duration of functional neutralizing antibodies against SARS-CoV-2 can vary greatly and it is important to monitor this at an individual level.

Waning antibodies do not always translate into decreased immunity, and people with low levels of neutralizing antibodies may still be protected from Covid-19 if they have a robust T-cell response. The study also found that patients from all groups, including those who did not have detectable neutralizing antibodies, had sustained T-cell immunity 6 months after the infection. These results add to evidence that people with acquired immunity may have differing levels of protection to emerging SARS-CoV-2 variants. More importantly, those who have had and recovered from a Covid-19 infection still stand to benefit from getting vaccinated [19].

Immunity needs to confer protection against severe disease and mortality as well as infection and mild symptoms of the disease. Notably, correlates may differ depending on the endpoint used [20]. It is estimated that neutralizing antibody levels required for protection against severe disease are about six times lower than the level required to protect against any symptomatic infection [21]. If there is no detectable antibody response after vaccination, the vaccines may still offer protection through cellular immunity. Although this may be true in some cases, cellular immune responses and antibody responses often correlate to some extent [22]. Antibody responses do not seem to correlate with overall protection against asymptomatic infection. There is no one level on any of the binding or neutralizing antibody assays used that provides full protection against the virus [23].

4.3 *A snapshot of what we know and do not know*

People have had natural immunity for over 1 year at the time of writing and the reinfection rate is high among them (when compared to vaccinated individuals). Vaccines were introduced in 2021, giving about 7–8 months of follow-up data, which show that the breakthrough infection rate after vaccination is low.

Infections and vaccinations generate memory B cells and T cells [24]. Memory B cells are activated upon reinfection and manufacture high levels of antibodies from plasma cells in the bone marrow, even years after initial exposure [24]. T cells, in the form of either CD4+ cells or CD8+ cells, attack and kill pathogens, such as viral particles. Thus far, T-cell responses to Covid-19 vaccines are strong and long-lasting, even against different variants. Data to date suggest that individuals previously infected with SARS-CoV-2 who are subsequently vaccinated exhibit the best vaccine response and may not need a booster vaccine, but individuals not previously infected may require additional doses, if at all [24].

4.4 *Vaccine-induced immunity*

When the first Covid-19 vaccine study results were announced in late 2020, the efficacy of the vaccinated candidates sent waves of jubilation among the scientific community. Since then, more than 3.7 billion Covid-19 vaccine doses have been administered worldwide [25], and we have also seen the rise of new coronavirus variants like the Delta and Omicron, which can partially evade the protective immunity conferred not only by natural acquired immunity but also by vaccines.

The terms efficacy and effectiveness are sometimes used interchangeably, in the context of vaccines, but it is important to understand the difference between the two. Efficacy is the measure of how much disease the vaccine prevents, and possibly transmission, under ideal and controlled circumstances. Effectiveness refers to how well the vaccine performs in the real world — including against new variants, and in people who may have been excluded from clinical trials, such as elderly individuals, those with comorbidities, or those taking immunosuppression drugs [26].

The impact of effective reproduction number Rt/Re on vaccine effectiveness is well reported [15] — the effects of any Covid-19 vaccine are highly dependent on the effective reproductive number of the virus (Rt or Re) at the time a vaccine is deployed. Rt functions in part as a proxy for the success of efforts to promote widespread, sustained adherence to risk mitigation strategies, such as masking, physical distancing, and limitations to large gatherings. When Rt is comparatively low (1.5), indicating that viral circulation is being controlled through non-pharmaceutical measures, vaccines with low efficacy (25%) are capable of producing larger reductions in the fraction of infections and deaths than vaccines with much higher efficacy (75%), which are introduced at times when Rt is significantly higher (2.1). Furthermore, the additional benefit of a vaccine with 25% vs. 75% efficacy very much depends on the background Rt; in cases of outbreak control (Rt ≤ 1.5), a vaccine with 25% efficacy might well have a substantive impact. Even the effects of a vaccine with 90%–95% efficacy rely heavily on the background Rt at the time of its introduction [15]. The US Centers for Disease Control and Prevention advises that even after being fully vaccinated, people should continue to mask up and socially distance in public places in part because they could still unknowingly become infected and, although asymptomatic, may transmit SARS-CoV-2 to people who have not yet received/completed their vaccine shots [27]. Transmission by infected asymptomatic vaccinees could provide an opportunity for more virulent variants to spread [27].

The reduced cross-protection to novel variants (Table 1), heterogeneity of infection-acquired immunity (Table 2), and waning immunity to vaccines with lower initial efficacy (Table 3) are significant concerns, given that control measures are likely to rely on population immunity effects and the resulting case counts, hospitalizations, and fatalities. This is a critical factor for SEA as the vaccination rates are low and slow, the infection rates are high, and the variants are rapidly spreading, pushing the threshold for reaching population immunity higher [21].

Predictive modeling techniques based on vaccine efficacy data have been used by scientists to estimate the durability and duration

Table 3. Waning effect of vaccines (based on initial efficacy).

Vaccine	Initial Efficacy	Days to 70% Efficacy	Days to 50% Efficacy
Pfizer-Moderna	95%	200	250
Sputnik-V	92%	150	225
Convalescent	88%	120	210
Bharat Biotech	80%	51	149
AD26 Johnson & Johnson	67%	—	52
Choxl Astra Zeneca	62%	—	48
Coronovac SinoPharm	50%	—	—

of immune protection conferred by seven different vaccines over time. The results suggest that the immediate protection following vaccination is predictive of a more durable response (Table 3). Consequently, the protection offered by vaccines with >90% immediate efficacy could last about 8 months, whereas vaccines with under 70% initial efficacy might lose their potency in about 2 months [21].

4.5 *Covid-19 therapeutics*

It is now fairly well established that much of the damage to the lung and the organs is not directly attributed to the virus but rather as a consequence of an overactive immune response, termed cytokine storm [28]. Early effective treatment of Covid-19 can help avert progression to more serious illness, especially for patients at high risk of disease progression and severe illness, with the additional benefit of reducing the burden on healthcare systems [29].

The spectrum of medical therapies to treat Covid-19 is growing and evolving rapidly (Figure 6). Remdesivir is the first of the few anti-viral medications approved by the Food Drug and Administration (FDA) to treat Covid-19. The approval was based on findings that hospitalized patients who got remdesivir recovered faster [29].

Monoclonal antibody treatment has been authorized for emergency use to treat mild-to-moderate Covid-19. Researchers are also

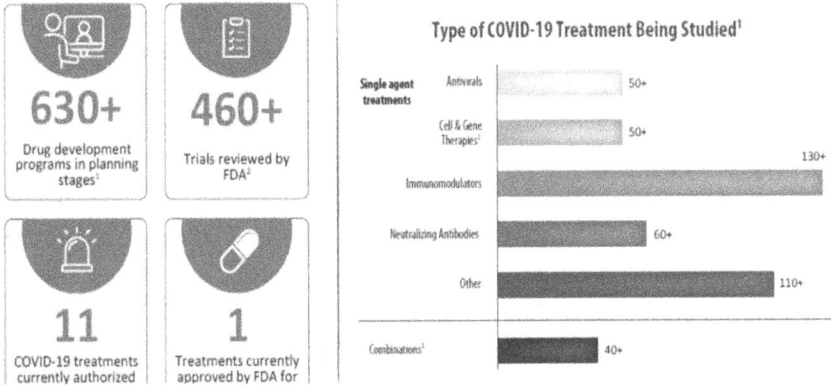

Figure 6. An overview of drugs and therapeutics under development, under review and approved by the FDA.

testing older medications (that are typically used to treat other conditions) to see whether they are also effective for Covid-19 [29].

Immunomodulators, used for the treatment of arthritis and other autoimmune diseases, are being tested in Covid-19 patients. A number of novel therapeutics (e.g., monoclonal antibodies) are available under emergency use authorization (EUA) for early outpatient treatment. Trials to assess the potential effectiveness of these therapeutics in outpatients at high risk of disease progression are ongoing [29].

5. Outlook for the Future and Recommendations

The threat of a prolonged Covid-19 pandemic, with recurrent waves in some countries, is the main risk to the outlook, as it would require protracted caution and containment measures, with consequent economic turmoil. The spread of the virus depends on contacts, which depend on economic activity; conversely, economic activity depends on the spread and trajectory of the virus [30]. Most of the SEA countries managed to flatten the first epi curve to save millions of lives in 2020. "Lockdown fatigue" and prolonged unemployment contribute to a desire to resume economic activity. The only way to flatten the subsequent waves is to identify the Covid-19 infection and reduce the intermingling of the infectious and the susceptible population. Failure in identifying the cases lays the groundwork for possible surge; hence, at this point, countries have no choice but to execute lockdowns. Lockdowns greatly impact the economy by halting normal and routine business operations. Scaling up testing capacity to quarantine the infectious population while continuing vaccination may be the most cost-effective option rather than implementing costly lockdowns.

5.1 *Testing*

Testing can reduce the severity of lockdowns required to achieve a given reduction in the spread of disease [30]. It helps hold down the medium- and long-term public health impact, cumulative death toll, and economic scarring [30]. The estimated economic benefits and costs of such measures are of the order of 4–15:1. Net benefits rise further if one additionally monetizes deaths averted using a statistical value of life [30].

Centre for Economic Policy Research studies reveal that stringent government lockdown measures involve a trade-off between health benefits (e.g., lower infections and/or mortality) and economic benefits (e.g., lowering economic output) [31].

Testing had positive indirect effects on growth and perhaps even positive direct effects. By allowing countries to relax shutdowns without compromising on containment, testing could have indirectly contributed to about a 0.6% boost in growth [31]. By encouraging greater confidence in people to step out and engage in economic activity, testing could have attained the 0.6% growth [31].

Testing is only as good as its frequency, strategy, scale, and compliance. If probable or suspected asymptomatic people are missed because only symptomatic people get tested, then the benefits of such a strategy will be lost. The "silent spreaders" will go undetected, perpetuating the chain of transmission in mass congregations and social events as mobility increases [31].

In the wake of a slow and low vaccination rate and high transmission, the best way to safely reopen the economy is to establish a

Table 4.   SMART testing framework.

Framework		Potential Scenarios
S	Surveillance	Immune surveillance for gauging community immunity and genomic surveillance to identify variants
M	Monitoring	Healthcare workers and essential services workforce
A	Asymptomatic screening	Pre-events, gatherings, public places, and probable and suspect contacts of confirmed COVID-19 cases
R	Return to work testing	Frequency of testing based on risk assessment stratification and the prevalence in the community
T	Triage and diagnosis	Symptomatic cases

comprehensive testing regimen for Covid-19. The Surveillance, Monitoring, Asymptomatic screening, Return to work testing, Triage and diagnosis (SMART) testing framework helps realize a safe return to economic activity with genomic and immune surveillance, monitoring of essential workforce and frontline healthcare workers, asymptomatic screening for events and entertainment, and return-to-work testing to keep the workplace safe and testing of symptomatic cases for triage and clinical management (Table 4).

5.2 *Vaccination*

Vaccination, when performed at a rapid pace across large populations, is a very powerful tool to reduce not only the severity of the disease in individuals but also the virus transmission in the community. The benefits of any Covid-19 vaccine — whether highly, moderately, or modestly efficacious by the clinically defined outcome — will depend at least as much on how swiftly and broadly it is implemented and the epidemiological environment into which it is introduced.

The benefits of any Covid-19 vaccine will decline substantially in the event of manufacturing or deployment delays, significant vaccine hesitancy or greater epidemic severity. The vaccine roll-out strategy needs to be not only fast but also across the region. This is the only way to win the race against variants and to fully reopen sectors such as travel and tourism, which account for over 8.4% of gross domestic product (GDP) in some SEA countries [32]. As long as the virus is active somewhere in the region, the likelihood and risk of new virus variants are high, which will mean that some borders will have to remain closed, restraining mobility. Vaccines will be central in attaining community immunity and thus prevent local spread due to case importation. Although vaccine-specific characteristics are fixed, countries can productively intervene concerning the contextual considerations that would increase the benefits of a vaccine upon its introduction. Fully vaccinating 20% of the population is estimated to have the same effect as closing down public transport and all-but-essential workplaces. Fully vaccinating 50% of the population would have a larger effect than simultaneously applying all forms of containment policies in their most extreme form (closure of workplaces, public transport, and schools; restrictions on travel and gatherings; and stay-at-home requirements) [33]. For SEA countries, relaxing existing containment policies would be expected to raise the GDP by about 4–5% [33]. Quick vaccination would thus help limit the extent to which containment policies need to be escalated in future epidemic waves, providing significant benefits in terms of both fewer infections and safer and stronger return to economic activity [33]. Even with a stronger supply, some SEA countries are to ramp up national vaccination programs quickly. It will be a double tragedy for the region if the problem shifts from too few vaccines to too many to be used effectively. Much of the region will need ongoing donor assistance to overcome vaccine hesitancy, expand vaccination services, and solve "last-mile" logistical and storage challenges [34].

6. Conclusion

The region is facing an unprecedented health threat, which is triggering economic consequences, revealing geopolitical vulnerabilities, and suggesting further societal challenges ahead. In addition to the dangers to public health, the pandemic and the resulting lockdowns and shutdowns could have long-lasting effects on people and societies.

There is an urgent need for health officials to invest greater financial resources and to redouble efforts to promote public confidence in Covid-19 testing and vaccines and to encourage continued adherence to other mitigation approaches, even after vaccination. Expanding efforts to identify and reach high-risk areas and groups is critical for stopping small, localized hotspots from spiraling into national and regional emergencies. An effective communication campaign and clear protocols for hospitalization and management of cases can also help reduce the strains on the healthcare system. The length and depth of the current economic crisis will depend on solving the healthcare crisis. Access to vaccines, tests, and treatments for everyone who needs them is the only way out — this is a test for regional and global cooperation.

References

[1] Phua, J., Faruq, M. O., Kulkarni, A. P. *et al.* (2020). Asian analysis of bed capacity in critical care (abc) study investigators, and the Asian critical care clinical trials group. Critical care bed capacity in Asian countries and regions. *Critical Care Medicine,* **48**(5), 654–662.

[2] Population of South-Eastern Asia (2021). — Worldometer (worldometers.info). https://www.worldometers.info/world-population/south-eastern-asia-population/, accessed 1 August 2021.

[3] Chookajorn, T., Kochakarn, T., Wilasang, C. *et al.* (2021). Southeast Asia is an emerging hotspot for COVID-19. *Nature Medicine.* https://doi.org/10.1038/s41591-021-01471-x.

[4] Thailand braces for COVID-19 spike after Songkran holiday. https://asia.nikkei.com/Spotlight/Coronavirus/Thailand-braces-for-COVID-19-spike-after-Songkran-holiday, accessed 22 July 2021.

[5] IHME (2021). COVID-19 results briefing, The South-East Asia Region, July 14.

[6] Hasell, J., Mathieu, E., Beltekian, D. *et al.* (2020) A cross-country database of COVID-19 testing. *Scientific Data,* **7**, 345.

[7] Kronbichler, A., Kresse, D., Yoon, S., Lee, K. H., Effenberger, M., and Shin, J. I. (2020). Asymptomatic patients as a source of COVID-19

infections: A systematic review and meta-analysis. *International Journal of Infectious Diseases*, **98**, 180–186.

[8] Kuster, A. C. and Overgaard, H. J. (2021). A novel comprehensive metric to assess effectiveness of COVID-19 testing: Inter-country comparison and association with geography, government, and policy response. *PLoSOne*, **5**, 16(3): e0248176.

[9] https://www.moh.gov.sg/, accessed 10 August 2021.

[10] Southeast Asia and COVID-19 vaccines explained. https://southeastasiacovid.asiasociety.org/southeast-asia-and-covid-19-vaccines-explained/, accessed 1 August 2021.

[11] Rella, S. A., Kulikova, Y. A., Dermitzakis, E. T. *et al.* (2021). Rates of SARS-CoV-2 transmission and vaccination impact the fate of vaccine-resistant strains. *Scientific Reports*, **11**, 15729.

[12] Phipps, S. J., Grafton, R. Q., and Kompas, T. (2020). Robust estimates of the true (population) infection rate for COVID-19: A backcasting approach. *Royal Society Open Science*, **7**, 200909.

[13] Understanding the journey to herd immunity. https://www.path.org/articles/understanding-journey-herd-immunity/, accessed 25 July 2021.

[14] Fine, P., Eames, K., and Heymann, D. L. (2011). Herd immunity: A rough guide. *Clinical Infectious Diseases*, **52**(7), 911–916.

[15] Can we predict the limits of SARS-CoV-2 variants and their phenotypic consequences? https://assets.publishing.service.gov.uk/government/uploads/system/uploads/attachment_data/file/1007566/S1335_Long_term_evolution_of_SARS-CoV-2.pdf, accessed September 2021.

[16] Haddad, D., John, S. E., Mohammad, A. *et al.* (2021). SARS-CoV-2: Possible recombination and emergence of potentially more virulent strains. *PLoSOne*, **16**(5), e0251368.

[17] Planas, D., Veyer, D., Baidaliuk, A. *et al.* (2021). Reduced sensitivity of SARS-CoV-2 variant Delta to antibody neutralization. *Nature*, **596**, 276–280.

[18] From the frontlines: understanding herd immunity. https://www.lung.org/blog/understanding-covid-herd-immunity, accessed 22 August 2021.

[19] Chia, W. N., Zhu, F., Ong, S. W. X. *et al.* (2021). Dynamics of SARS-CoV-2 neutralising antibody responses and duration of immunity: A longitudinal study. *Lancet Microbe*, **2**(6), e240–e249. Erratum in: *Lancet Microbe*, May 2021; **2**(5): e179.

[20] Krammer, F. (2021). A correlate of protection for SARS-CoV-2 vaccines is urgently needed. *Nature Medicine*, **27**, 1147–1148.

[21] Khoury, D. S., Cromer, D., Reynaldi, A. *et al.* (2021). Neutralizing antibody levels are highly predictive of immune protection from symptomatic SARS-CoV-2 infection. *Nature Medicine*, **27**, 1205–1211.

[22] Grifoni, A., Weiskopf, D., Ramirez, S. I. *et al.* (2020). Targets of T cell responses to SARS-CoV-2 coronavirus in humans with Covid-19 disease and unexposed individuals. *Cel,.* **181**(7), 1489–1501.e15.

[23] Feng, S., Phillips, D. J., and White, T. (2021). Correlates of protection against symptomatic and asymptomatic SARS-CoV-2 infection. https://www.medrxiv.org/content/10.1101/2021.06.21.21258528v1. full.pdf.

[24] Palm, A.-K. E. and Henry, C. (2019). Remembrance of things past: Long-term B cell memory after infection and vaccination. *Frontiers in Immunology*, **10**. https://www.frontiersin.org/article/10.3389/fimmu. 2019.01787.

[25] Coronavirus (COVID-19) Vaccinations — Statistics and Research — Our World in Data, accessed 1 August 2021.

[26] What is the difference between efficacy and effectiveness? https:// www.gavi.org/vaccineswork/what-difference-between-efficacy-and-effectiveness, accessed 2 August 2021.

[27] Rubin, R. (2021). COVID-19 vaccines vs variants — Determining how much immunity is enough. *JAMA*, **325**(13), 1241–1243.

[28] Sinha, P., Matthay, M. A., and Calfee, C. S. (2020). Is a "cytokine storm" relevant to COVID-19? *JAMA, Internal Medicine*, **180**(9), 1152–1154.

[29] Testing for Covid-19: A way to lift confinement restrictions. https:// www.oecd.org/coronavirus/policy-responses/testing-for-covid-19-a-way-to-lift-confinement-restrictions-89756248/, accessed 2 August 2021.

[30] Atkeson, A., Droste, M., Mina, M., and Stock, J. (2020). Economic benefits of COVID-19 screening tests. National Bureau of Economic Research Working Paper, No 28031.

[31] Islamaj, E., Le, D. T., and Matto, A. (2021). Lives versus livelihoods during the COVID-19 pandemic: How testing softens the trade-off. *Covid Economics*, 80, 9 June, CEPR Press.

[32] Southeast Asia faces GDP loss of 8.4% in 2021 as COVID-19 roils tourism. SEADS (adb.org), accessed 8 August 2021.

[33] Turner, D., *et al.* (2021). The tortoise and the hare: The race between vaccine rollout and new COVID variants. OECD Economics

Department Working Papers, No. 1672, OECD Publishing, Paris, https://doi.org/10.1787/4098409d-en.

[34] Southeast Asia and COVID-19 vaccines explained. https://southeastasiacovid.asiasociety.org/southeast-asia-and-covid-19-vaccines-explained/, accessed 2 August 2021.

https://doi.org/10.1142/9789811255151_0009

Chapter 9

Two Viral Pandemics, a Century Apart and a Potential "Twindemic" on Collision Course in Southeast Asia

Mohan Ravuru*, Yong Poovorawan[†],
Carmenchu Echiverri-Villavicencio[‡],
Rontgene M. Solante[§], and Aw Tar Choon[¶,‖]

*Abbott Rapid Diagnostics, Singapore
[†]Center of Excellence in Clinical Virology, Department of Pediatrics
Faculty of Medicine, Chulalongkorn University, Thailand
[‡]Department of Infectious Disease, St. Luke's Medical Center
Department of Medicine, Section of Infectious Disease
St. Luke's Global City, The Philippines
[§]Philippine College of Physicians
Philippine Society for Microbiology and Infectious Diseases
Infectious Diseases Society of America (IDSA)
San Lazaro Hospital, Quiricada Street, Santa Cruz,
Manila, Philippines
[¶]Duke-NUS Graduate Medical School, Singapore
Changi General Hospital, Singapore

[‖]Corresponding author.

This chapter covers:

- Historical perspective on the impact of the Spanish flu pandemic in Asia between 1918 and 1920.
- An overview of similarities and differences between Covid-19 and influenza.
- Lessons from the evolution of influenza and Covid-19.
- Timeline, history, and brief overview of emerging viral infectious disease outbreaks in Asia in the 21st century.
- The uncertainties and unpredictability around the collision course of influenza and Covid-19.
- Potential public health consequences of influenza and Covid-19 co-infection.
- The need for outbreak preparedness and key recommendations.

1. Introduction

Emerging infectious diseases due to novel pathogens have significantly increased over the past few decades, due to changes in various environmental, biological, socioeconomic, and political factors. Trends in globalization, international travel and trade, and human mobility have all extended the human reach and increased the pace at which infectious diseases spread. The path toward globalization of the Asian economy, in particular, is strewn with many obstacles — population explosion, deforestation, ecological erosion, loss of natural habitat, human and animal migration, and rapid urbanization, to name a few [1]. Almost 200 million people have moved to urban areas in East Asia during the first decade of the 21st century [2].

Subsistence farming, livestock, and proximity of domestic and non-domestic animals due to lack of space allow for mixing of different species, including humans, creating a favorable environment for zoonotic outbreaks and disease transmission [2]. Tropical regions, rich in host biodiversity, offer a large pool of zoonotic pathogens, greatly increasing the possibility of novel ones to emerge [1].

Southeast Asia has been an epicenter of EID over the last decade, including those with pandemic potential. These diseases have exacted heavy toll on health and economy in the recent past [3]. The majority of diseases are zoonotic (many of wildlife origin), suggesting the practices at the human–animal interface may facilitate the likelihood of spillover of zoonotic pathogens into humans. It also underlines the importance of biodiversity as a source of EID [1]. The potential for the prevention and mitigation of disease outbreaks in the region is noteworthy, as evidenced by recent response to the Covid-19 pandemic.

The Covid-19 pandemic has created significant imbalance to our way of life, diminishing host dominance, and turned the spotlight back on human behavior, sanitation, and hygiene. Across Southeast Asia, most public health agencies are still grappling with the health and economic devastation caused by recurrent waves of Covid-19 infections due to the emerging SARS-CoV-2 variants and slow rollout of Covid-19 vaccines. Healthcare systems are weakened and stretched to capacity, and healthcare workers are overworked and in a state of pandemic fatigue. The efforts being taken to mitigate the spread of the coronavirus seemed to have helped in keeping the seasonal flu at bay. The southern hemisphere has already witnessed two winter seasons without flu cases.

Going forward, there are significant potential public health risks associated with an overlap of Covid-19 and seasonal influenza outbreaks in the collision course of circulating SARS-CoV-2. The population immunity to Covid-19 has not yet reached a steady state while the two low-profile flu seasons have left the populations largely unprotected against future strains of flu. Low flu vaccine and drug uptake in Asia are compounding the problem further.

2. Historical Overview of Influenza Pandemic of 1918 — "The Spanish Flu"

Between August 1918 and March 1919, while World War I was ongoing, the world experienced a catastrophic outbreak of a highly contagious respiratory disease called the Spanish influenza [4]. The flu was first detected in March 1918 in US troops training at Camp Funston, Kansas. The 1918–1919 pandemic quickly circled the globe, and most of humanity felt the effects of the flu as it followed trade routes and shipping lines. The Great War, in its twilight years and during demobilization, exacerbated the rapid diffusion of the pandemic. Outbreaks swept through North America, Europe, Asia, Africa, Brazil, and the South Pacific, partly through war-time military mobilization, infecting one-third of the world's population and claiming over 50 million lives.

Wartime censorship meant that the US and European media were not permitted to report on the outbreaks. Spain, however, was neutral in the conflict. The country's newspapers reported so extensively on the disease that it soon became known as the Spanish flu.

The death toll outnumbered the war casualties. There were no effective diagnostics, drugs, or vaccines at that time to combat the disease. Most of its infected victims experienced aches and fever which worsened over days, sometimes abruptly. There was widespread fear and panic. As a public health strategy, patients were urged to stay home for several extra days upon the detection of relapses among those who resumed their normal routines too quickly. At a critical stage of its spread, the infection prompted precautionary measures that bear striking resemblance to the current efforts at fighting Covid-19 [5,6]: authorities closed gathering places, such as theaters, cinemas, schools, places of entertainment, and public transport systems. Masks were distributed. Although the disease continued to spread to various parts of the planet, keeping people apart reduced the level of infection — if such isolation could be sustained [4].

The recorded statistics of influenza morbidity and mortality are likely to be a significant understatement. Limitations of these data can include non-registration, missing records, misdiagnosis, and non-medical certification, and may also vary greatly between locations. Further research has seen the consistent upward revision of the estimated global mortality of the pandemic, which a 1920s calculation put in the vicinity of 21.5 million [7]. A 1991 paper revised the mortality as being in the range 24.7–39.3 million. Research suggests that it was of the order of 50 million. However, it must be acknowledged that even this vast figure may be substantially lower than the real toll, perhaps as much as 100% understated [4].

The 1918 pandemic manifested as three distinct "waves," [8] with the first in the spring of 1918, the second in the fall of 1918, and the third in the winter of 1918–1919 (Table 1 and Figure 1).

The second wave was thought to be caused by a mutant, more virulent virus and spread by troop movements across Europe during World War I [9,10]. There was reluctance to impose control measures, since they would interfere with the war effort. Most of the deaths occurred with the second wave [11].

Table 1. The three waves of Spanish flu.

	Wave 1	Wave 2	Wave 3
Dates	Spring 1918	Fall 1918	Winter 1918–1919
Severity	Mild	Virulent	Less virulent
Deaths	50 million to 100 million, mainly young adults and pregnant women		
Mortality Rate	5%, up to 33% of isolated populations		

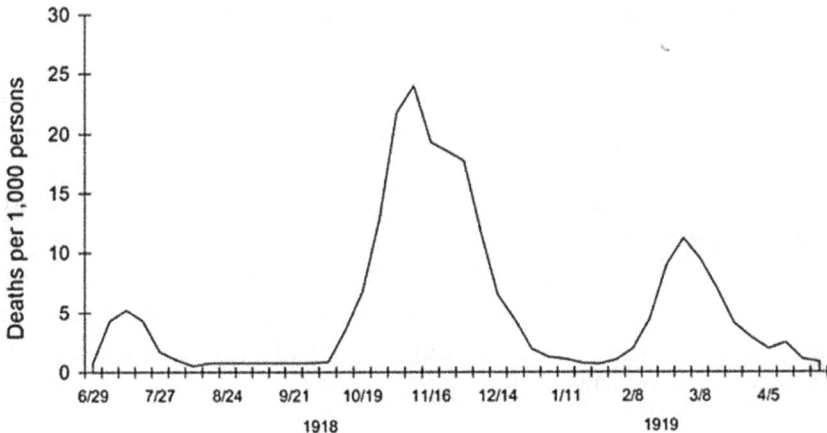

Figure 1. Three waves of death during the pandemic: Weekly combined influenza and pneumonia mortality, 1918–1919 [4].

Table 2. An overview of the estimates of mortality rates from the influenza pandemic, selected Asian countries, Fall wave 1918 [9].

Country	Total Deaths	Deaths per 1,000 Population
Indonesia	1.5 million	30.6
British Malaya	40,000	
Philippines	70,000–90,000	6.8–9.2
Thailand	80,223	
Other East and Southeast Asia	220,000–1.3 million	5–30.6
Southwest Asia	215,000–430.000	5–10
China	4.0–9.5 million	10–22.5
India	12.5–20 million	42–67
Japan	350,000	6.4
Whole continent, Asia	19–33 million	19.7–34.2

The influenza pandemic made its mark on Asian countries as well, although with vastly different effects in each of the Southeast Asian nations [12,13] (Table 2). An estimated 30 million deaths occurred in Asia, with India bearing the brunt of the devastation with over 15–20 million deaths, and Indonesia topped the Southeast Asian list with over 4 million deaths. The legacy of Spanish flu in Asia is substantial: the influenza viruses of 1957, 1968, and 2009 are all descendants of the H1N1 virus that caused the 1918 pandemic [10].

British Malaya: On a conservative estimate, within the months from June to November, the 1918 flu pandemic reached the shores of the colony in two waves, taking away a conservative estimate of 35,000–40,000 deaths. These figures dwarfed that of the more sensational SARS pathogen, which claimed 33 lives in Singapore and about 1,000 around the world [14].

Thailand: Influenza was initially reported in the south in October 1918, then spread throughout the Kingdom before subsiding in

March 1919. At the time, there were 17 administrative counties representing 73 provinces in Thailand with the combined total population of 8,478,566. The total number of influenza patients was 2,317,662, which resulted in 80,223 recorded deaths. The mortality rate was therefore approximately 1% of the total population [15].

Philippines: The cases were first noted among longshoremen and other laborers along the waterfront near Manila's ports, indicating that it had been brought in. Between June and December 1918, the Spanish flu epidemic resulted in 70,513 total number of deaths, with morbidity count at 40% of the total population [16].

Indonesia: Being the world's fourth most populous country in 1918, the most widely used estimate of mortality from that pandemic is 1.5 million. This number has been upwardly revised, taking Java and Madura, home to the majority of Indonesia's population into consideration, using additional data sources like population data from census. The new estimates suggest that, for Java alone, population loss was in the range of 4.26–4.37 million, or more than twice the established estimate for mortality for all of Indonesia [17].

3. Comparison of Influenza and Covid-19 and Key Inferences

As we are still in the midst of the current Covid-19 pandemic, it is hard to fathom the scope and after-effects of this public health crisis, but there are already some striking similarities as well as differences with the 1918 pandemic (Table 3).

- The SARS-CoV-2 and the H1N1 viruses were new to human populations, which means that there was no natural immunity to them. This may partially explain why the fatality rates of both diseases were significantly higher than the previous seasonal influenza and coronavirus outbreaks.
- The 1918 flu had multiple waves much like the current pandemic. Although the current situation is still developing, it is likely to mimic other pandemics. The second wave of the

Table 3. A comparison of the Spanish flu and Covid-19.

Pandemic	Spanish Flu	COVID-19
Virus	H1N1	SARS-CoV-2
Source	Avian (waterfowl)	Bats?
Intermediate host	Swine	Unknown
Origin	Military personnel, Fort Riley, Kansas	Wuhan, China
Year	Early March 1918	End December 2019
Period	1918–1919	2019–?
Affected groups	Children <5 yrs, Adults 20–40 yrs, Elderly >65 yrs	Initially in elderly with co-morbidities but to spread to all age groups
Case count	~500 million	>172 million by June 2021
Mortality	~50 million	>3.5 million by June 2021
Complications	Respiratory failure, MODS, Septic shock	Bronchopneumonia, pulmonary haemorrhage
Vaccine	None	Nine vaccines in use across the world and many more in the pipeline
Diagnostic test	None	Molecular, antigen and antibody tests available worldwide
Estimated Reproduction Number R0	2–4	
Mode of transmission	Direct contact, aerosol spread of respiratory droplets, contact with fomites, environmental surfaces	
Mode of entry	Mucous membranes of the mouth, eyes and nose	
Latent period and viral shedding	5–6 days. Similar patterns of viral shedding from infectious patients, and presumably comparable generation intervals.	
Dispersion parameter	Comparable dispersion parameter, k defined, which controls the variance in distribution of the number of secondary cases caused by a typical primary case. A smaller k value implies a bigger contribution to total infections from super-spreaders.	
Target organ	Lung	

Table 3. (*Continued*)

Pandemic	Spanish Flu	COVID-19
Containment and mitigation measures	Isolation, quarantine, personal hygiene, disinfectant use, closure of businesses, schools, public gatherings, travel restrictions, lockdowns	
Case fatality rate	Comparable case fatality rates (CFR) in some situations. It was conventionally accepted that the CFR for 1918–19 influenza was 2%. For Covid-19, the crude CFR shows a wide range, but covering 2%.	

Spanish flu pandemic was much more lethal than the primary wave and eerily enough, the second wave of Covid-19 caused more deaths than the first, particularly in South and Southeast Asia.

- SARS-CoV-2 is much more lethal than previously discovered coronaviruses because it so readily attacks human cells, especially the respiratory mucosa and lungs.

- SARS-CoV-2 is the largest single-stranded RNA genome (~30 kilobases, kb) among all RNA virus families and encodes about 29 proteins. This is three times the size of HIV or Hepatitis C, and twice the size of influenza virus genome. This enormous genetic diversity may allow it to recombine more quickly with other SARS-CoV-2 and develop into more problematic strains.

- Unlike many other viruses, SARS-CoV-2 also has a genetic proof-reading mechanism that inhibits mutations. This is probably why antiviral medications are less effective against SARS-CoV-2 because such drugs may induce mutations that blunt the lethality of the virus.

- Like the 1918 flu, Covid-19 produces a massive release of cytokines. This "cytokine storm" primarily targets lung tissue, resulting in pneumonia often followed by oxygen deprivation and death.

- Unlike Covid-19, which appears to hit the elderly and the ones with comorbidities the hardest, the Spanish flu struck primarily young adults. This may be why fear was so much greater among the general public and why lockdown measures may have been more palatable than they are now [6].

- In the case of both pandemics, there was no treatment at the time [6]. Despite intense effort around the world for vaccines and therapies for Covid-19, there is no treatment that lowers the viral load (although the medicine Remdesivir does appear to shorten hospital stays).
- Until a therapy is developed that prevents transmission or counters the effects of the SARS-CoV-2 virus, the primary defense is controlled and preventive human behavior.
- Like other coronaviruses, SARS-CoV-2 may adapt to target new species. It has been hypothesized that SARS-CoV-2 may have originated in bats/pangolins and migrated to humans.
- Studies show that the virus strain (H1N1) that caused the pandemic stayed back as the seasonal flu, and at times, merged with other types of flu (bird flu, swine flu, etc.) to create more dangerous strains — the outbreaks that happened in 1957 (H2N2 virus, Asian flu), 1968 (H3N2 virus, Hong Kong flu), and 2009 (H1N1, swine flu) were all contributed in part by the influenza virus.
- In summary, the virus strain (H1N1) that caused the influenza pandemic in 1918 never went away — it is still lingering in the background through its distant descendants, and people gained immunity over time to fight the virus. If the evolution of coronaviruses is any hint, this possibility is highly likely with SARS-CoV-2 as well.

4. 21st Century Viral Disease Outbreaks

The large outbreaks, since the start of 21st century (Table 4), have exposed the world's vulnerability to threats arising from new pathogens and have shown how humans inhabiting the planet make the emergence of new diseases more inevitable. Countries with high standards of living, robust healthcare systems, and sophisticated hospitals have not been spared from the onslaught of viral outbreaks [18]. The severe acute respiratory syndrome (SARS) in 2003 took its

Table 4.   Major viral disease outbreaks, timeline, and death toll.

Year	Name	Type/Intermediate Host (Pre-Human Host)	Number of Deaths
1889–1890	Russian Flu	Believed to be H2/N2 (Avian origin)	1 million
1918–1919	Spanish Flu	H1N1 virus/Pigs	40–50 million
1957–1958	Asian Flu	H2N2 virus	1.1 million
1968–1970	Hong Kong Flu	H3N2 virus	1 million
1981–present	HIV/AIDS	Virus/Chimpanzees	25–30 million
2009–2010	Swine Flu	H1N1 virus/Pigs	157,000–575,400 (upward revised numbers)
2002–2003	SARS	Coronavirus/Bats, Civets	770
2014–2016	Ebola	Ebola virus/Wild animals	11,000
2015–present	MERS	Coronavirus/Bats, camels	850
2019–present	Covid-19	Coronavirus-unknown (possibly Pangolins)	4.84 million (as of 7 Oct 2021)

Source: Compiled with data from CDC, WHO, and PAHO.

heaviest toll on wealthy urbanized nations and hurt economy and health. SARS spread most efficiently and exposed the weaknesses of public health systems [18]. In addition to human factors, environmental factors such as water, soil, mosquito vectors, and animals are also contributing to the outbreaks of viral diseases.

Severe Acute Respiratory Syndrome (SARS) 2002–2003: SARS is a respiratory disease characterized by dry cough, fever, headache, and body pain and is transmitted through droplets discharged from sneezing and coughing (Table 4). The first outbreak of the 21st century, SARS appeared in November 2002. It exploded rapidly to become an international health issue in March 2003. The World Health Organization (WHO) declared an international travel alert. It infected 8,098 people, caused 774 deaths, and precipitated travel bans in several countries. SARS spread mainly by flights to cities such as Singapore, Hong Kong, and Toronto. In all, it affected 29 countries and five continents. By early July 2003, WHO had announced an end to its spread. Containment policies followed case tracking, isolation, quarantine, the dissolution of mass gatherings, screening and testing of travelers, recommendations for improved personal hygiene, and barrier protection, and the containment operation successfully limited the outbreak [19].

Middle East Respiratory Syndrome (MERS) 2012: MERS is a viral respiratory disease caused by a novel coronavirus (Middle East respiratory syndrome coronavirus, or MERS-CoV) that was first identified in Saudi Arabia in 2012 (Table 4). Approximately 35% of reported patients with MERS-CoV infection have died. Although most of human cases of MERS-CoV infections have been attributed to human-to-human infections in healthcare settings, current scientific evidence suggests that dromedary camels are a major reservoir host for MERS-CoV and an animal source of MERS infection in humans. However, the exact role of dromedaries in transmission of the virus and the exact route(s) of transmission are unknown [20].

The Swine Flu 2009–2010: In 2009, the world was alerted to an outbreak of influenza, the swine flu (H1N1), which had purportedly spread from pigs to humans in Mexico (Table 4). Its origins were quickly traced to the town of La Gloria, which had witnessed cases of a severe respiratory illness since March 2009. By mid-March, about 60 of the village's inhabitants were reportedly ill with flu-like symptoms. By April 2009, 1,800 cases of swine flu had been recorded in Mexico along with several deaths. The numbers of suspected cases rose to 1,995, and by the end of the month, 149 victims had died. Tourists and business folks returning from Mexico facilitated the spread of the disease abroad. By late April, the US had confirmed 40 cases, Canada six, United Kingdom two, and Spain one, in addition to suspected cases in other countries.

The virus was found to be easily transmitted between humans, signaling its devastating potential. Many countries and governmental organizations issued prompt calls for emergency measures to prevent travel to and from infected regions. The WHO declared it a pandemic on 11 June 2009, which further heightened media interest and worry globally. In many countries, numerous private and public sector employees were alerted to safety and preventive steps. Schools and public places which experienced outbreaks were closed [21].

In April 2009, several countries announced embargos on imports of pork produced in Mexico and the US [21]. In 2009, the H1N1 virus, or swine flu, had an official death toll of 18,500. This was later revised upwards by *The Lancet* to between 151,700 and 575,400 deaths, which brings it close to seasonal flu, which accounts for between 290,000 and 650,000 deaths worldwide every year, according to the WHO [21].

The 21st century has already recorded more than 10 major epidemic or pandemic virus emergence events, including the ongoing and devastating Covid-19 pandemic (Figure 2A) [22]. Most of the major viral disease epidemics or pandemics in human populations, thus far, have been caused by coronavirus, alphavirus, myxovirus, filovirus, norovirus, and flavivirus family of viruses (Figure 2B) [22].

Occurrence of rapidly mutating viruses, emergence and reemergence of epidemics with increasing frequencies, and climate-sensitive

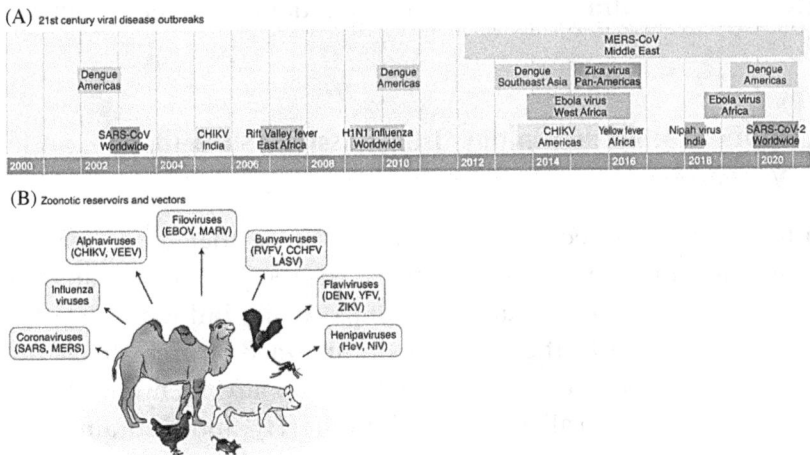

Figure 2. (A) Timeline of 21st-century viral outbreaks, from 2000 to the present day. Viral strains and the area of outbreak are indicated along with the timeline. (B) Animals, such as the ones shown, are zoonotic reservoirs or vectors for a number of virus families with pandemic potential [22].

vector-borne diseases are likely to increase over the years and the trends are likely to persist and possibly intensify, particularly in the Asia-Pacific region. Susceptible disease hosts, anthropogenic activities, and environmental changes contribute and trigger the "adaptive evolution" of infectious agents to thrive and spread into different ecological niches and to adapt to new hosts [23].

Although there has been substantial progress in recent years in the Southeast Asia region, which has seen reductions in deaths from HIV and malaria and an increase in tuberculosis treatment coverage, the region continues to bear a significant proportion of the communicable disease burden worldwide (Table 4). South Asia has the third largest HIV epidemic globally and the highest tuberculosis burden, accounting for more than a quarter of the global burden. The second highest incidence of malaria, amongst all WHO regions, occurs in the Southeast Asia region, and India bears the third-highest proportion of malaria cases globally. Malnutrition makes the Southeast Asian population particularly vulnerable to neglected tropical diseases (NTDs) alongside emerging infectious diseases from arbovirus infections, dengue, chikungunya, Japanese encephalitis, and the continuing concern of a pandemic influenza outbreak (Table 5).

5. Influenza: Epidemiology, Transmission, Surveillance, and Vaccinology

Influenza is an infectious respiratory disease that, in humans, is caused by influenza A and influenza B viruses. Both types can cause mild to severe illness in all age groups. While influenza A viruses infect humans and other animals, influenza B viruses affects only humans. Subtypes of type A influenza virus are identified by two antigenic proteins called hemagglutinin [H] and neuraminidase [N] on the surface of the virus. These proteins can change, or mutate, over time. Because these proteins can change, people can get influenza infections multiple times over their lifetime. An antigen "shift" (major change) creates a new influenza A virus with a new H, or H and N, that can cause a global epidemic if the virus can

Table 5. Summary of select emerging infectious diseases in Southeast Asia.

	Primary Transmission	Comments
Emerging diseases		
Avian influenza A H5N1	Zoonotic (close contact with poultry)	325 reported cases, 224 deaths in Indonesia, Vietnam, Thailand, Cambodia, Laos, and Myanmar
Pandemic influenza A H1N1 (2009)	Respiratory	5,290 reported cases, eight deaths in all 10 countries
SARS	Respiratory	331 reported probable cases, 44 deaths in Singapore, Vietnam, Thailand, Malaysia, and Indonesia
Nipah virus	Zoonotic (close contact with pigs)	First known human cases in Malaysia; 276 cases, 106 deaths in Malaysia and Singapore
Re-emerging diseases		
Chikungunya fever	Vector-borne	Endemic in many Southeast Asian countries; re-emerged in Singapore (2008), Malaysia (2007), Thailand (2009), and Indonesia (2010)
Dengue fever	Vector-borne	Originated in Southeast Asia; 398,340 cases and 1,596 deaths in 2008 with high burden in Indonesia, Vietnam, Thailand, Malaysia, the Philippines, Myanmar, and Cambodia; estimated 253,000 DALYs lost in 2004
Japanese encephalitis	Vector-borne and zoonotic	Only 68 reported cases in Thailand 2009; estimated 243,000 DALYs lost in 2004
Rabies	Zoonotic (bite or scratch from rabid animal)	587 cases and deaths in 2009 in Indonesia, the Philippines, Vietnam, Myanmar, and Thailand

(Continued)

Table 5. *(Continued)*

	Primary Transmission	Comments
HIV/AIDS	Sexual, injecting drug use, vertical	High adult HIV prevalence (more than 0.5%) in Thailand, Cambodia, and Myanmar, with more than 200,000 HIV-positive people in Thailand, Vietnam, Indonesia, and Myanmar; estimated 2,952,000 DALYs lost in 2004
Streptococcus suis	Zoonotic (close contact with pigs)	Case reports from Thailand and Vietnam
Leptospirosis	Zoonotic (skin contact with urine of rodents)	5,697 cases and 83 deaths in 2009 with high burden in Thailand and reported cases in Indonesia and Myanmar
Drug-resistant diseases		
MDR tuberculosis	Respiratory	2,332 cases in 2008; high-burden countries are the Philippines, Myanmar, Indonesia, and Thailand
XDR tuberculosis	Respiratory	Detected in Myanmar, the Philippines, Singapore, Thailand, and Vietnam
MDR *Plasmodium falciparum* malaria	Vector-borne	Documented on Cambodia's border with Thailand

Notes: SARS = severe acute respiratory syndrome. DALYs = disability-adjusted life-years. MDR = multidrug resistant. XDR = extensively drug resistant.

spread easily among people and if most people do not have immunity against it. This happened most recently in 2009 when the novel H1N1 influenza virus appeared and led to a major pandemic [24].

Typically characterized by annual seasonal epidemics, sporadic pandemic outbreaks involve influenza A virus strains of zoonotic origin. Influenza A viruses that infect humans mainly consist of two strains (H1N1 and H3N2) [24]. Seasonal influenza epidemics cause approximately 3 to 5 million cases of severe influenza and about 290,000 to 650,000 respiratory deaths each year globally. The Asia-Pacific region is believed to have a similar burden of influenza to countries with temperate climates, but is considered to be an important source of new viruses and global influenza epidemics due to its large and highly interacting human and animal populations [25].

5.1 *Influenza transmission and surveillance zones*

The WHO Influenza Transmission Zones are geographical groups of countries, areas, or territories with similar influenza transmission patterns (Figure 3). Asia covers five such transmission zones. The timing of epidemics varies between these transmission zones, as does the number of outbreaks per year and the extent of inter-epidemic transmission [24].

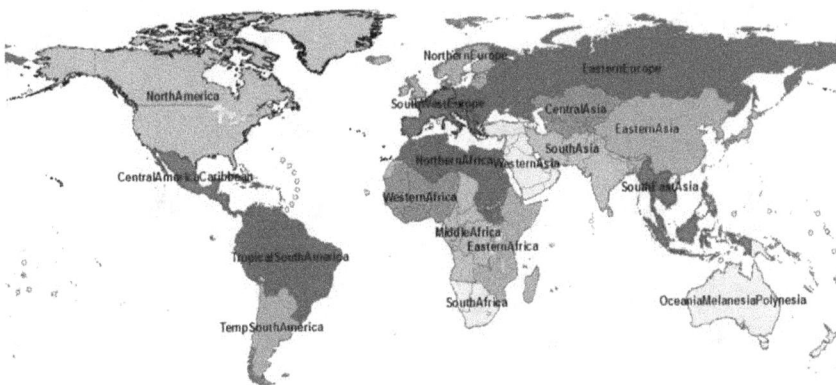

Figure 3. WHO Influenza Transmission Zones as well as the list of countries, areas, or territories by zone.

Two key factors that determine the timing and intensity of an influenza epidemic are climate and population immunity to the circulating strain. In tropical/sub-tropical Southern and Southeast Asian countries, influenza infections are reported throughout the year, with generally two outbreaks per year. The primary peak is between May and October for most of these countries but this is not synchronized. In the Western, Central, and Eastern Asian transmission zones, influenza infections are largely confined to the winter season, with peaks between December and March. Outbreak timing within each zone seems generally synchronized though there is some evidence of an East to West spread within the Western Asia transmission [24].

5.2 *Highlights of the global influenza surveillance update* [26]

Globally, despite continued or even increased testing for influenza in some countries, influenza activity remained at levels lower than expected for this time of the year. In the temperate zones of the southern hemisphere, influenza activity has remained at the low inter-seasonal levels (Figure 4).

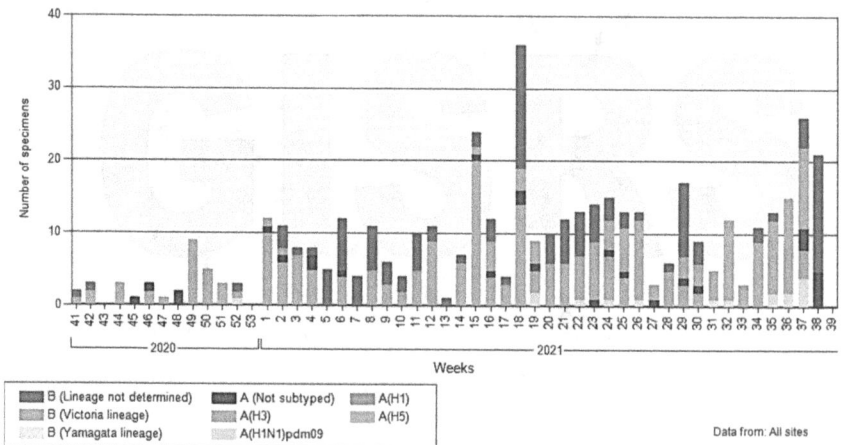

Figure 4. Number of specimens positive for influenza by subtype (Southern Hemisphere).

Source: FluNet (www.who.int/flunet).

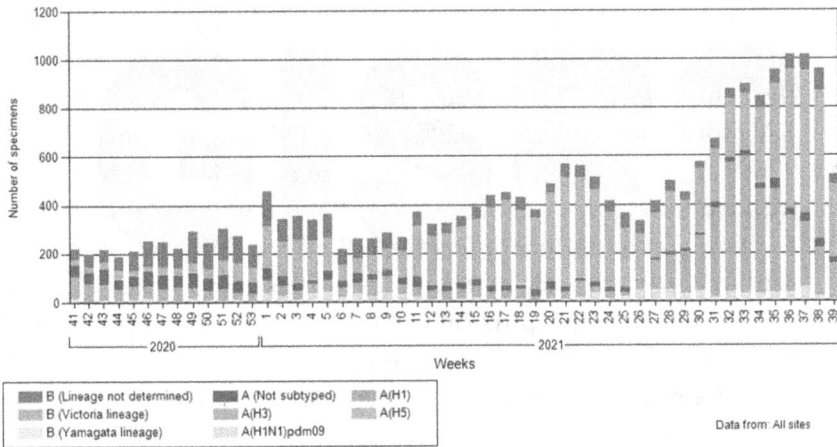

Figure 5. Number of specimens positive for influenza by subtype (Northern Hemisphere).

Source: FluNet (www.who.int/flunet).

- In the temperate zones of the northern hemisphere, influenza activity remained at inter-seasonal levels (Figure 5).
- In the Caribbean and Central American countries, sporadic influenza B virus detections were reported in some countries.
- In tropical South America, one influenza A detection was reported in Peru in this period.
- In tropical Africa, a few influenza detections of predominately influenza A were reported in some countries in Western, Middle, and Eastern Africa.
- Worldwide, influenza A and B viruses were detected in similar proportions.
- National Influenza Centers (NICs) and other national influenza laboratories from 88 countries, areas or territories reported data to FluNet for the time period from 30 August 2021 to 12 September 2021 (data as of 2021-09-24 07:02:37 UTC).
- The WHO GISRS laboratories tested more than 275,940 specimens during that time period; 1,884 were positive for influenza viruses, of which 808 (42.9%) were typed as influenza A and 1,076 (57.1%) as influenza B.

- Of the sub-typed influenza A viruses, 54 (7.3%) were influenza A(H1N1)pdm09 and 686 (92.7%) were influenza A(H3N2). Of the characterized B viruses, 973 (99.8%) belonged to the B-Victoria lineage and 2 (0.2%) to the B-Yamagata lineage.
- The current influenza surveillance data should be interpreted with caution as the ongoing Covid-19 pandemic has influenced, to varying extents, health-seeking behaviors, staffing/routines in sentinel sites, as well as testing priorities and capacities. The various hygiene and physical distancing measures implemented by countries to reduce SARS-CoV-2 virus transmission have likely played a role in reducing influenza virus transmission [26].

5.3 Influenza surveillance update from Asia

In Southern Asia, influenza detections of predominately influenza A(H3N2) and influenza B continued to be reported across several countries. In Southeast Asia, sporadic influenza A(H3N2) detections were reported in the Philippines (Table 6).

Influenza A and B are co-circulating in the region, however, the majority of cases reported from week 37, 2020 to week 35, 2021 have been influenza B (Figure 6).

6. Current State of Play and the Overlap "Twindemic" Scenario

The virulence of the circulating strains, transmission dynamics, pre-existing population immunity, and the age-groups most prone to infection play a role in severity and incidence of influenza each year [27]. Unfortunately, these very factors are at play with the ongoing Covid-19 pandemic and the convergence of these two pathogens and infections creates uncertainty around the potential consequence of this collision course. The emergence of delta variants, recurrent waves of transmission, the slow roll-out of Covid-19 vaccines in Southeast Asia, the resulting toll on human health and economy, the pandemic fatigue, strained health systems and healthcare workers, are creating a cloud of uncertainties about the future.

Table 6. Virological surveillance summary (22 September 2021).

Country (most recent week of report)	Total Number of Specimens Processed	Total Number of Influenza Positive Specimens
Australia (34)	65,488	3
Cambodia (32)	3,208	0
China (34)	426,304	7,391
Fiji (4)	222	
Japan (33)		4
Lao People's Democratic Republic (35)	2,105	146
Malaysia (33)	2,073	2
Mongolia (31)	306	0
New Caledonia		
New Zealand		
Papua New Guinea		
Philippines (32)	391	48
Republic of Korea		
Singapore (34)	1,897	1
Viet Nam (30)	497	39

Source: WHO, FluNet.

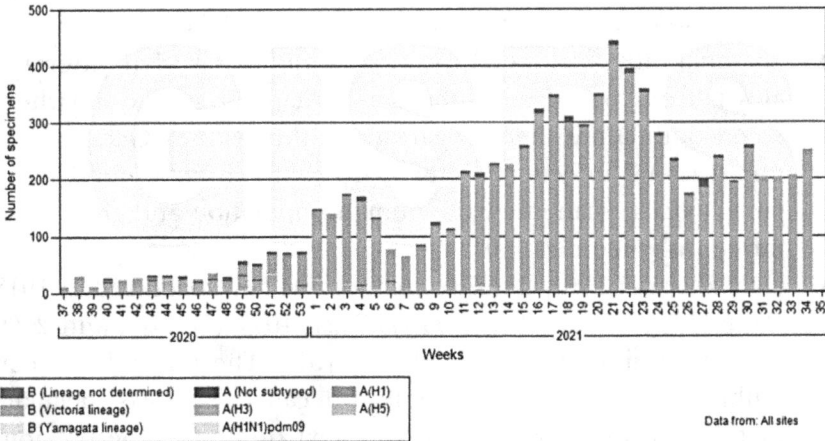

Figure 6. Number of specimens positive for influenza subtype, Western Pacific region, week 37, 2020 to week 35, 2021.

Source: WHO, FluNet.

- Covid-19 infection control strategies to help prevent the spread of disease in community settings have aligned with those used for other common respiratory viral infections such as influenza.
- Robust preventive measures like international travel restrictions, wearing masks, hand hygiene, and physical distancing may have also helped to prevent influenza transmission.
- Despite these mitigation measures, Covid-19 continued to spread, demonstrating that SARS-CoV-2 is much more contagious than the influenza virus [28].
- During a typical season, about 20%–30% of the population is exposed to the flu. If two full seasons are nullified, it would leave a significant proportion of population susceptible and vulnerable to infection, due to lack of immunity, notwithstanding the cumulative effect of low flu vaccine and drug uptake [25]. The magnitude of the impact is unfathomable.
- Influenza vaccines are adapted and formulated every year to match the circulating strains, as the viruses mutate [29]. Furthermore, influenza vaccine efficacy is suboptimal and is dramatically low in the case of an antigenic mismatch between the vaccine and the circulating virus strain. Antiviral agents are available for prophylaxis and therapy, but the uptake of flu vaccines and drugs is very limited in Southeast Asia.
- Seasonal influenza is cyclic in nature and this is what differentiates it from pandemic influenza, which can spread anywhere across both hemispheres regardless of the weather. Occasionally, non-seasonal infection events can occur, whereby novel influenza A viruses can enter the human population and give rise to influenza epidemics [30].
- Over the past 100 years, five such events have occurred in 1918 (H1N1), 1957 (H2N2), 1968 (H3N2), 1977 (H1N1), and 2009 (H1N1), claiming millions of lives [31]. The interval between outbreaks has reduced to about a decade. Scientists speculate that we are long overdue for the next outbreak (the previous one was in 2009).

- Those at risk for severe influenza infection are children, pregnant women, elderly, those with underlying chronic medical conditions, and those with co-morbidities such as compromised immunity, diabetes, obesity and cardiovascular disease [31]. The background baseline prevalence of the comorbid conditions is relatively higher in Asia.
- The regional differences in Covid-19 transmission, policy measures to limit spread, and differences in reopening stages across Southeast Asian nations would mean it will be important to monitor seasonal influenza activity concurrently with Covid-19.
- The co-circulation of influenza and Covid-19, both of which cause respiratory illness, may be on a trajectory for collision. The apparition of a "twindemic" — two epidemics at the same time — looms large in Southeast Asia and could potentially place an additional burden on vulnerable populations and healthcare systems that are already stretched thin because of the Covid-19 pandemic.
- Detecting whether a person has flu or coronavirus based on clinical signs and symptoms is difficult. Rapid flu and Covid-19 screening and short turnaround time to results can help with management and treatment of both viruses and they can eliminate anxiety for patients and healthcare personnel.
- Covid-19 and influenza co-infections had significantly different rates of incidence in Wuhan, China during two distinct time periods of the Covid-19 pandemic and that co-infection with influenza B virus was more likely to result in a poor prognosis [32].
- Experimental cell culture and mouse models have shown that an influenza A infection led to the promotion of increased SARS-CoV-2 infectivity and viral load resulting in increased lung damage [33].
- Some people may get infected with multiple viruses simultaneously, which could make symptoms more severe. Pathogens may influence one another with both positive and negative effects, adding complexity to clinical diagnosis, treatment, and patient management.

7. The Need for Outbreak Preparedness and Key Recommendations

The Covid-19 pandemic continues to have a major impact on health-care, social, and economic systems throughout Asia. As the clinical and epidemiological features of Covid-19 have many parallels with influenza, it is important to ensure optimal management of both respiratory diseases as we anticipate their continued co-circulation and co-infection with Covid-19. In particular, there is a need to ensure that effective surveillance and diagnostic capacities are in place to monitor these and other respiratory viruses, as this will underpin decisions on the appropriate clinical management of the respective diseases.

The Southeast Asian region has long been recognized as an important source of novel influenza viruses and for the generation of seasonal influenza viruses, followed by their global circulation. The emergence and then subsequent spread of the avian influenza H5N1 virus in domestic poultry and the associated human infections in late 2003, the Hong Kong flu in 2009, and emergence of the avian H7N9 virus in 2013, reinforce the importance of ongoing surveillance initiatives to understand and control influenza in the region.

The current substantial uncertainties, novelty of the evolving evidence, limited understanding of SARS-CoV-2 and viral interactions, co-infections, super-infections, and secondary infections dictate that absolute conclusions of certainty about "future outbreaks or recurrent waves" cannot be made. Future preparedness and planning for outbreaks should be informed by regular monitoring, robust surveillance, the adaptability of response-based evidence, and scenario modeling. The complex pathophysiology that arises from dual infections of SARS-CoV-2 and influenza viruses underlines the importance of vigilant detection and diagnosis.

As such, we propose a series of key recommendations for stakeholders, public health authorities, primary care physicians, and surveillance bodies that will help mitigate the combined risks of concurrent influenza epidemics and the Covid-19 pandemic.

- Regardless of how well flu shots match up with the circulating strains, flu vaccination is going to be extremely important.
- Prioritize influenza vaccination programs, particularly vaccinating those at high risk of developing complications, including pregnant women, the elderly, children, and people with underlying health issues.
- The symptoms of flu and Covid-19 — with the exception of anosmia (loss or decrease of the sense of smell) — are very similar, this necessitates to test for both flu and SARS-CoV-2.
- Influenza A co-infection is not an uncommon occurrence in Covid-19 patients, and leads to significantly higher hyperinflammation and longer disease course. With the ongoing flu season and gradual relaxation of Covid-19 restrictions in many parts of Asia, rates of co-infection are likely to increase despite ongoing vaccination, because immunization of a sufficient proportion of the population takes time.
- Combined testing for both viruses at decentralized settings and clinics that regularly review influenza like illness (ILI) and severe acute respiratory illness (SARI), should be made widely available. Screening of high-risk patients for seasonal flu and Covid-19 should be considered a high priority.
- There is an imminent need for a stockpile of combined screening tests, so people on the frontlines can differentiate those two viruses, treat those that need to be treated for influenza, and also alert public health officials if it is Covid-19, in terms of quarantine and contact tracing.

It is likely that the increased use of emerging technologies such as digital and mobile tools for testing, tracing, tracking, and treating, along with telemedicine will permanently change our approach to managing infectious disease. The existing pharmaceutical strategies and non-pharmacologic interventions, will ensure that we achieve a holistic approach to the global public health measures needed to deal with the combined threat of influenza and Covid-19. Ensuring that this approach is optimal will be key as we move from a reactive pandemic response toward preparing for the long-term management of the remarkable clinical burden associated with these respiratory pathogens.

References

[1] Morand, S., Jittapalapong, S., Suputtamongkol, Y., Abdullah, M. T., and Huan, T. B. (2014). Infectious diseases and their outbreaks in Asia-Pacific: Biodiversity and its regulation loss matter. *PLoS ONE*, **9**(2), e90032.

[2] World Bank Group. 2015. East Asia's changing urban landscape: Measuring a decade of spatial growth. Washington, DC: World Bank. https://openknowledge.worldbank.org/handle/10986/21159.

[3] Coker, R. J., Hunter, B. M., Rudge, J. W., Liverani, M., and Hanvoravongchai, P. (2011). Emerging infectious diseases in Southeast Asia: Regional challenges to control. *Lancet*, **377**(9765), 599–609.

[4] Taubenberger, J. K. and Morens, D. M. (2006). 1918 Influenza: The mother of all pandemics. *Emerging Infectious Diseases*, **12**(1), 15–22. doi: 10.3201/eid1201.050979.

[5] WHO COVID-19 Weekly Epidemiological Update Edition 54, published 24 August 2021. Weekly epidemiological update on COVID-19 — 24 August 2021 (who.int), accessed 27 August 2021.

[6] He, D., Zhao, S., Li, Y., Cao, P., Gao, D., Lou, Y., and Yang, L. (2020). Comparing COVID-19 and the 1918–19 influenza pandemics in the United Kingdom. *IJID*, **98**, P67–P70.

[7] Johnson, N. P. and Mueller, J. (2002). Updating the accounts: Global mortality of the 1918–1920 "Spanish" influenza pandemic. *Bulletin of the History of Medicine*, Spring; **76**(1), 105–115.

[8] Centers for Disease Control and Prevention. 1918 pandemic influenza: Three waves. Reviewed May 11, 2018. Accessed August 26, 2021. https://www.cdc.gov/flu/pandemic-resources/1918-commemoration/three-waves.htm

[9] Taubenberger, J. K. (2005). Chasing the elusive 1918 virus: Preparing for the future by examining the past. In: Knobler, S. L, Mack, A., Mahmoud, A., and Lemon, S. M. (eds.) *The Threat of Pandemic Influenza: Are We Ready?* Workshop Summary. Institute of Medicine, National Academies Press, pp. 69–89.

[10] Taubenberger, J. K. and Morens, D. M. (2010). Influenza: The once and future pandemic. *Public Health Reports*, **125**, Suppl 3, 16–26.

[11] Roos, D. (2020). Why the second wave of the 1918 Spanish flu was so deadly. *History.com*. March 3, 2020. Updated March 30, 2020. https://www.history.com/news/spanish-flu-second-wave-resurgence, accessed April 9, 2020.

[12] https://earth.org/data_visualization/pandemic-map-the-spanish-flu/, accessed 1 August 2021.

[13] Patterson, K. D. and Pyle, G. F. (1991). The geography and mortality of the 1918 influenza pandemic. *Bulletin of the History of Medicine*, Spring, **65**(1), 4–21. PMID: 2021692.

[14] Liew, K. K. (2007). Terribly severe though mercifully short: The episode of the 1918 Influenza in British Malaya. *Modern Asian Studies*, **41**(2), 221–252. https://www.jstor.org/stable/4132351

[15] Ratchakitchanubegsa (1919). **36**; July 27, pp. 1193–1202. http://www.ratchakitcha.soc.go.th/DATA/PDF/2462/D/1193.PDF, accessed 1 June 2021 (in Thai).

[16] Gealogo, F. A. (2009). The Philippines in the world of the influenza pandemic of 1918–1919. *Philippine Studies*, **57**(2), 261–292, www.jstor.org/stable/42634010, accessed 26 August 2021.

[17] Chandra, S. (2013). Mortality from the influenza pandemic of 1918–19 in Indonesia. *Population Studies*, **67**(2), 185–193. doi:10.1080/00324728.2012.754486.

[18] How the 4 biggest outbreaks since the start of this century shattered some long-standing myths. https://www.who.int/news/item/01-09-2015-how-the-4-biggest-outbreaks-since-the-start-of-this-century-shattered-some-long-standing-myths, accessed 6 October 2021.

[19] 2009 H1N1 Pandemic (H1N1pdm09 virus). https://www.cdc.gov/flu/pandemic-resources/2009-h1n1-pandemic.html, accessed 7 October 2021.

[20] Middle East respiratory syndrome coronavirus (MERS-CoV). https://www.who.int/news-room/fact-sheets/detail/middle-east-respiratory-syndrome-coronavirus-(mers-cov), accessed 7 October 2021.

[21] Influenza A (H1N1) outbreak. https://www.who.int/emergencies/situations/influenza-a-(h1n1)-outbreak, accessed 7 October 2021.

[22] Meganck, R. M. and Baric, R. S. (2021). Developing therapeutic approaches for twenty-first-century emerging infectious viral diseases. *Nature Medicine*, **27**, 401–410. doi: 10.1038/s41591-021-01282-0.

[23] Priyadarsini, S. L., Suresh, M., and Huisingh, D. (2020). What can we learn from previous pandemics to reduce the frequency of emerging infectious diseases like COVID-19? *Global Transit*, **2**, 202–220.

[24] Young, B. E. and Chen, M. (2020). Influenza in temperate and tropical Asia: A review of epidemiology and vaccinology. *Human Vaccines & Immunotherapeutics*, **16**(7), 1659–1667.

[25] El Guerche-Séblain, C., Caini, S., Paget, J. *et al.* (2019). Epidemiology and timing of seasonal influenza epidemics in the Asia-Pacific region, 2010–2017: Implications for influenza vaccination programs. *BMC Public Health*, **19**, 331. doi: 10.1186/s12889-019-6647-y.

[26] https://www.who.int/teams/global-influenza-programme/surveillance-and-monitoring/influenza-updates/current-influenza-update, accessed 9 October 2021.

[27] Kamigaki, T., Chaw, L., Tan, A. G., Tamaki, R., Alday, P. P., Javier, J. B., Olveda, R. M., Oshitani, H., Tallo, V. L. *et al.* (2016). Seasonality of influenza and respiratory syncytial viruses and the effect of climate factors in subtropical–tropical Asia using influenza-like illness surveillance data, 2010–2012. *PLoS One*, **11**: e0167712. doi: 10.1371/journal.pone.0167712.

[28] Covid-19 and the flu. https://asm.org/Articles/2020/July/COVID-19-and-the-Flu, accessed 9 October 2021.

[29] How flu viruses can change: "Drift" and "Shift". https://www.cdc.gov/flu/about/viruses/change.htm, accessed 9 October 2021.

[30] Krammer, F., Smith, G. J. D., Fouchier, R. A. M. *et al.* (2018). Influenza. *Nature Reviews Disease Primers*, **4**, 3. doi: 10.1038/s41572-018-0002-y.

[31] Saunders-Hastings, P. R. and Krewski, D. (2016). Reviewing the history of pandemic influenza: Understanding patterns of emergence and transmission. *Pathogens*, **5**(4), 66. doi:10.3390/pathogens5040066.

[32] Bai, L., Zhao, Y., Dong, J., *et al.* (2021). Coinfection with influenza A virus enhances SARS-CoV-2 infectivity. *Cell Research*, **31**(4), 395–403. doi: 10.1038/s41422-021-00473-1.

[33] Stowe, J., Tessier, E., Zhao, H., *et al.* (2021). Interactions between SARS-CoV-2 and influenza, and the impact of coinfection on disease severity: A test-negative design [published online ahead of print, 2021 May 3]. *International Journal of Epidemiology*, doi: 10.1093/ije/dyab081.

Chapter 10

Leading in the New Normal

Karin Sixl-Daniell

Singapore University of Social Sciences, Singapore

The years since early 2020 have brought tremendous change to the whole world. Covid-19 and its consequences have led to unprecedented interruptions affecting organizations and individuals alike, be it in Asia or the globe. Millions of deaths were brought upon mankind. Lockdowns, circuit breakers, shutdowns, and the like took a toll on business life from the company as well as the employee perspectives, with companies having to at least temporarily shut down across the globe and employees receiving no or a reduced salary. Supply chains were and are still interrupted. Further disruptions due to war and further diseases are likely to prolong this phase of a New Normal, leading to new requirements for leadership in times of uncertainty, fear, and anxiety.

New approaches to the working life add to new requirements for leadership as well. While authoritarian top-down approaches may have worked in the past, research has shown that there is a shift to more quality of life and individualism [1]. The workforce shows a tendency to an increased emphasis on work–life balance (or "life–work balance"), and lower birth rates in many countries point toward a problem with overaging societies and, simultaneously, fewer people active in the workforce, resulting in a lack of talent. The lack of skilled workers and talent is a phenomenon that can be observed all over the globe which, together with the emphasis on more work–life balance and individualism, leads to new and bigger challenges in and for leadership.

1. The Concept of Leadership

A leader can be appointed, such as by holding a formal position in the company. Other leaders may act as leaders because the other group members perceive this person as the most influential in their group. This type of leadership is therefore not related to position, but is formed through communication. These are people who are verbally involved, informing, inquiring about others' opinions, initiating new ideas, and being firm but not intransigent [2].

The concept of power is related to leadership because power is a component of the process of influence. Power is expressed through influencing the attitudes and thoughts of others. Many people see the exercise of power as part of leadership. However, research with a focus on power in leadership is limited. Exercising power through coercion is a special case of the power available to leaders. Coercion often involves the use of threats and punishment. Leadership by coercion must be considered separately, because coercion serves the pursuit of one's own interests — this also forms the distinction from leadership.

In many areas, leadership is similar to management. Management also involves exerting influence, working with other people, and achieving goals. Nevertheless, there are differences: the theories of leadership can be traced back to Aristotle, while management had its beginnings with the Industrial Revolution. The primary function of management is planning, organizing, hiring, and controlling. Kotter [3] described the central function of management as ensuring order and stability, while leadership, on the other hand, focuses on change and movement as its primary function.

While traditionally, leadership was equaled to management, differences become clear and hence a move from a purely mechanistic and transactional nature of management (pay for work) to a different step in leadership became necessary.

2. Developments in Leadership

While a mechanistic and autocratic approach like for Taylor or Fayol in the early 20th century was the norm, various approaches to leadership were developed over the years. These ranged from leadership styles such as autocratic, democratic, and laissez faire (Lewin), to Weber's addition of a bureaucratic style, to Tannenbaum and Schmidt's Leadership Continuum, showcasing further differences between leadership styles. Blake and Mouton developed the Managerial Grid which focuses on leadership approaches along two axes labeled people-centered and task-centered. The combination of the positions based on the two axes would showcase an approach to leadership which could range from "impoverished" (for those not focusing on tasks nor people) to "country club" (for those focusing on people but not tasks) or "team management" (for those focusing on tasks and people). Such leadership obviously requires an involved leader who focuses on more than one dimension in their work.

Hersey and Blanchard developed an approach they labeled *Situational Leadership* which requires leaders to adjust their leadership behavior based on the respective follower's readiness and abilities. Hence, according to them, a differentiation between Telling, Selling, Participating, and Delegating is necessary.

These approaches already show how a move from the abovementioned transactional nature of work toward an approach that looks beyond the obvious (pay for work) started taking place.

In the New Normal, leading in the old ways will not prove successful and keywords such as Authentic Leadership, Servant Leadership, Empathetic Leadership, Agile Leadership, and Transformational Leadership have been widespread.

Authentic Leadership has been repeatedly discussed as in times of the New Normal, an authentic leader is needed. Someone who walks the talk and showcases a what-you-see-is-what-you-get approach; someone who is self-aware and self-reflected; someone who takes in feedback and is honest. The importance of authenticity could be seen clearly in numerous statements and at numerous occasions by business and political leaders alike during the pandemic; equally, the lack of but need for authenticity could be seen clearly in statements and at occasions by business and political leaders alike (e.g., Covid-19 parties at No. 10 Downing Street; leaders not wearing masks while the public is mandated to do so; leaders driving hundreds of kilometers to visit relatives during a lockdown).

Servant Leadership is about sharing power, putting people and their needs first, and thereby leading as a "servant" to reach organizational goals while not adhering to old, transaction-based concepts. Greenleaf, who coined the term in 1970, wrote:

> "The servant-leader is servant first... It begins with the natural feeling that one wants to serve, to serve first. Then conscious choice brings one to aspire to lead. That person is sharply different from one who is leader first, perhaps because of the need to assuage an unusual power drive or to acquire material possessions... The leader-first and the servant-first are two extreme types. Between them there are shadings and blends that are part of the infinite variety of human nature. The difference manifests itself in the care taken by the servant-first to make sure that other people's highest priority needs are being served. The best test, and difficult to administer, is: Do those served grow as persons? Do they, while being served, become healthier, wiser, freer, more autonomous, more likely themselves to become servants? And, what is the effect on the least privileged in society? Will they benefit or at least not be further deprived?" [4].

Servant leaders inspire others to go beyond the obvious, beyond what is expected because of their concern for others, contributing to overall success and goal achievement.

Empathetic Leadership focuses on the importance of actually showing and living empathy. During the pandemic, this has become even more important as hundreds of millions of people were affected by changes in their employment and/or paycheck status. Empathy in the workplace has risen to new heights as understanding the needs and feelings of others has become a necessity in order to ensure employees remain in the organizational realm. This empathy has already also shown increased organizational performance as employees feel valued and understood and at the same time feel a certain bond to an organization that was understanding in time of need and did not simply opt to lay off people in order to save costs. Once the businesses restarted, such organizations had a distinct competitive advantage as they had the necessary manpower available to get restarted available — as opposed to other organizations who let employees go and now have trouble rehiring, leading to inability to get the business engine running again.

Agile Leadership is based on agile methods in software development (self-organizing teams) and, as the name implies, focuses on an agile mindset. Static and fixed mindsets in silos will not work in the New Normal and adaptiveness, autonomy, nimbleness, and adaptability are needed. Organizations are not seen as static and organized in silos; rather, self-organized teams are at the front as organizations are viewed as living systems. Such systems are seen as dynamic while stable and can prosper in rapidly changing environments that could be seen during the pandemic. Quick changes were necessary in order to adapt: creativity and flexibility as well as redesigning (or doing away with) hierarchies and business models were needed to adapt to and survive in the new environment. Given the necessity to act quickly, nimbleness was needed. This nimbleness and agility will also be needed in the New Normal as organizations across the globe have learned to embrace agile approaches. Those not embracing agile approaches will no doubt have competitive disadvantages.

Transformational Leadership is centered on the four Is — Inspirational Motivation, Idealized Influence, Individual Consideration, and Intellectual Stimulation — to transform followers' approaches to work. These four Is ensure that followers are motivated to perform at unexpected levels, leading to superior organizational performance.

Inspirational Motivation encompasses setting and communicating a vision as well as adequately setting goals that act as an inspiration, require dedication and effort to achieve, but are doable. Both intrinsic as well as extrinsic aspects of motivation can be seen here.

Idealized Influence refers to a leader acting as a role model; often, followers try to emulate such leaders. This aspect of transformational leadership focuses on leaders "walking the talk" and showcasing traits followers try to emulate because of the leader's charisma. While in general seen as positive, this aspect may be problematic when applied in political settings (e.g., dictators) or cults.

Individual Consideration discusses the importance of adequate genuine attention and consideration given to followers to ensure their development. Mentoring is as much part of Individual Consideration as are carefully selected tasks to be delegated to followers to help them in their development.

Intellectual Stimulation is another central point in Transformational Leadership. Followers are encouraged to be creative, use intellectual stimuli, and not remain in fixed mindsets that tend to conform to the status quo. Instead, thinking out of the box is encouraged as is innovativeness — which in turn makes an error culture necessary where errors can be made and learned from.

Transformational Leadership is not to be seen as the antidote to transactional leadership as there are aspects of transactional leadership also in transformational leadership (after all, employees do get paid in return for their work), but rather as an approach going far beyond mere transactional approaches.

Crises, however, also demand quick action, and some authoritarian aspects can be also found in the discussion, leading to further development such as *Paradoxical Leadership*: A leader should be able to handle seemingly paradox or opposing approaches and integrate them to ensure effective leadership. This would refer to competing demands, e.g., followers' individual needs in parallel to organizational needs to exert authority and power over employees.

3. The New Normal and (Constant) Change

Companies in the New Normal face constant change. However, change often creates confusion, fear, and chaos. Such changes can refer to individual parts of organizations, but can also affect the entire organization. The goal now is to manage these changes as effectively and efficiently as possible, which is why the term change management — and with this also change leadership — came into being.

If an organization's environment evolves but its organizational structure and strategy remain the same, there may be a continuous deterioration of its competitive position over time. This is even more so the case in the New Normal, with changes in quick succession becoming the norm. If an organization does not adapt to these changes in the environment and its competitors, it will fall behind in competition and perish in the medium or longer term.

To deal with external change, an organization must adapt internally. It needs an adapted strategy, business model, and possibly also new products or services. Covid-19 showed this need to adapt at various levels in a striking manner.

However, there may also be reasons for change within the organization. Due to growth — especially in the founding phase of an organization — and as a result of an increasing number of employees, organizational design may need to be adapted and organizational development comes into play. Differentiations in product or service design also require adjustments to the organization. Depending on the markets served — local to national, international to global — further challenges can arise, including but not limited to organizational culture and cross-cultural aspects.

If an organization successfully follows a certain pattern for a long time, its behavior may become entrenched and complacency may set in. Organizations and their leadership sometime no longer feel the need to learn and attempt to repeat the old patterns in new market situations instead of adapting. However, this usually leads to a decline in success, as the examples of Nokia, Blackberry, or Kodak have shown.

Again, in the New Normal, such complacencies are even more ill placed and dangerous. Adequate leadership is required to navigate such rough seas.

When changes are imminent, projects dealing with them often experience a number of phases: An initial phase of surprise is followed by a phase of denial (state of denial), which in turn is followed by a kind of valley of tears. This is usually followed by an acceptance phase, which in turn is followed by a phase of experimentation, another of realization, and a final phase of integration. While this is the case in most change projects, it could also be seen in the pandemic and, the longer the pandemic prevailed, an additional "change fatigue" factor could be seen.

The goals of change leadership and organizational development are (among others) as follows:

- Improving the speed of response to changes, be it internal or external changes.
- Increasing flexibility to meet customer requirements.
- Developing and maintaining core competencies as strategic competitive advantages.

These goals also place high demands on an organization's employees who must continually adapt over time. Leadership has to steer all this, with HRM being supportive with its activities and sub-processes. By planning personnel requirements, the newly needed competencies can be recruited or (further) developed through training and education. By ensuring an adequate corporate culture open to new learnings, creativity, innovation, and empowerment, a leader has a significant role to play and is thus an essential dimension for and in managing and leading change.

Change becomes a constant (Heraclitus). Thus, the competence for change management is transformed from an exceptional case to a normal, often even essential task in and for the organization in the New Normal.

4. The Human Side of Leading Change

Every person reacts differently to uncertainty. Every person reacts differently to change. Some people perceive change as motivating, while others fear any change. Big changes in the environment and one's life such as during the pandemic can become problematic. Organizations face issues, as problems and challenges for one person would not only be multiplied by the people affected but, given the interactions between people, rise exponentially. If one takes these interpersonal effects of changes into account as well, it becomes clear that a plethora of issues can ensue.

Simply put, it is easier to avoid changes than to face and implement them. However, organizations have to deal with changed and changing environments in the New Normal and adapt to these in order to survive. For example, change may be necessary to improve and/or to survive (e.g., new processes, design, culture, knowledge base, and capabilities). The attitude in organizations has long been that change occurs sporadically and only when necessary in order to solve problems. In the meantime, and in particular during the time of the Covid-19 pandemic, it has been recognized that this is not the case and that change must be continuous in order to be successful and able to survive. Change management must be seen holistically and encompass all stakeholders. A successful change process must take into account diverse ideas and needs of different groups in an organization and integrate them into the management process.

If change is necessary, why is it so often met with strong resistance?

Generally speaking, resistance is shown when it would lead to subjectively felt "costs" (e.g., changes in behavior patterns and comfort zone), which then leads to minimizing these "costs" by opposing the changes. In organizations, this resistance is practically always found when there are changes in processes or procedures, etc. This resistance occurs for a number of reasons, some of which are briefly discussed here.

Short-term thinking is one of them. Most individuals find it extremely difficult to resist or delay gratification. Similarly, most prefer the present state of (often mistakenly assumed) comfort because gratification follows only at a later stage. While this gratification only comes later, the work necessary for it is required right away and associated with costs in terms of effort. With the potential fruits of the efforts far away and not tangible, individuals may find it particularly difficult to stay on track for changes as short-term thinking kicks in.

Another reason why individuals resist change is *self-interest*. Most people assess changes based on the effect these changes will or could have on *themselves* ("What's in it for me?") and not on the effect the changes will or could have on the *organization or society*. If changes are not viewed as positive, people tend to oppose them.

Both people and animals are afraid of the unknown. According to O'Toole [5], people prefer situations "with the devil they know than with the devil they don't know". *Fear and anxiety* are some of the most powerful factors when it comes to resistance to change as fear of the unknown and uncertainty play a huge role when people make decisions.

Habits are another area of potential reasons to oppose changes. It is easier to remain in habits because these habits are familiar and perceived as comfortable. Habits are hard to break, and to try new ways of working requires getting out of that comfort zone. Questions such as "Do we really have to change this process? Why?" and "Why can't I keep this exactly the way I've always done it?" are often raised along with comments such as "But why should we change, we have always done it this way!" The pandemic made it clear to many individuals that "we have always done it this way" may not be the way forward — particularly not with leading organizations.

Finally, *lack of self-confidence* is another theme to mention here. A new job setting, new technologies and new work processes may require different abilities and skill sets. Hand in hand with this, new ways of thinking and attitudes may also be required. This may be daunting for some. A fear of failure and of being seen as incompetent and lacking the necessary skills and abilities is often there and can be overwhelming.

Leading in the New Normal requires awareness of these points and the willingness to lead people in and through changes. Authentic, empathetic, and agile leadership is needed to work and navigate through various situations successfully while remaining sharp and on point with observations, walking the talk and acting as a role model.

5. Leading (through) Change in the New Normal

Change processes and their management and leadership are complex processes that do not allow for a one-dimensional view if they are to be successful. Various approaches try to represent change processes in a model-like and schematic way in order to obtain a simplified picture and to be able to act accordingly. These models include, inter alia, the approaches of Nadler and Tushman, Lewin, Kotter, Kanter, the ADKAR model, and McKinsey's 7S.

However, they usually refer to planned change. Naturally, an adaptation needs to happen if one is confronted with unplanned change. Organizational Culture is a powerful lever for managing change. A strong, positive organizational culture is linked with better organizational performance — and this shows also in times of change. In the New Normal, this becomes even more important.

Planned change has its limits, as the corporate environment often develops very dynamically. Even solidly prepared change projects can be outdone by reality, as organizations worldwide have seen since early 2020. Change in organizations therefore requires not only planning but also an aspect of improvisation, which, however, concerns details rather than the fundamental development of an organization. The already mentioned leadership approaches including Servant Leadership, Authentic Leadership, Empathetic Leadership, Transformational Leadership, as well as Agile Leadership are all part of organizational development and organizational well-being in the New Normal.

Change can no longer be planned as a rare event, an exception, but has become a regular in the New Normal. Adaptation to changing conditions can no longer be postponed until a future date, but needs to be carried out without delay.

One model of managing and leading change was developed by Harvard Business School Professor John Kotter who expanded Kurt Lewin's change model from three to eight stages. Kotter observed the following typical mistakes in the management of successful organizations in a dynamic environment:

- Too much complacency is tolerated.
- The creation of a sufficiently strong leadership coalition fails.
- The power of vision is underestimated.

- Lack of communication of the vision as even with an appropriate vision, managers sometimes forget that it is of absolute importance to repeat it relentlessly.
- Obstacles blocking the new vision are allowed (resistance to change).
- Quick successes are not planned, i.e., short-term thinking and the need for gratification are not seen.
- Victory is declared too early.
- Changes are not anchored in the corporate culture.

This can lead to new strategies not being implemented consistently, acquisitions not achieving the expected synergies, restructuring measures being both too time-consuming and cost-intensive, cost reduction programs not being effective, etc.

In order to avoid these negative effects, Kotter proposed the following eight steps for change management:

- Create a sense of urgency.
- Form a powerful guiding coalition.
- Develop a vision and strategy.
- Communicate the vision of change.
- Empower people to act on the vision.
- Ensure quick wins.
- Consolidate successes and initiate further changes.
- Anchor new approaches in the culture.

While very handy and applicable in practice, this model, as all the other models mentioned, was developed prior to the Covid-19 pandemic and hence looks more at leading *planned* change. The New Normal, however, often requires leading in *unplanned* change situations.

How can leadership in the New Normal act to navigate the rough seas that unexpectedly have been presenting themselves since 2020 and will continue to do so in the future? A possible approach could cover the following points:

1. Being a proactive leader, not a reactive one.
2. Showcasing the need for change while remaining empathetic.
3. Ensuring organizational politics are thought of with both formal as well as informal leaders on board.
4. Decision-making as much as possible free from the clouds of perceptual errors.
5. Deciding on the vision and showing the direction and the goal — using this as a guiding star.
6. Walking the talk.
7. Being transparent.
8. Proactively and constantly communicating to avoid rumors and manage expectations.
9. Actively soliciting feedback from stakeholders and taking it into consideration for the direction, the goals, and any potential adjustments of said direction and/or goal.
10. Appreciating inputs and the people involved in change efforts.
11. Working on the organizational culture to become (and remain) successful.
12. Ensuring an adequate error culture.
13. Practicing self-awareness and self-reflection.
14. Ensuring to be and remain on track for success — the original track or a potentially adjusted one. If necessary, adapting the course or even changing direction.
15. Developing adequate measures to showcase success (or lack thereof) of such changes.
16. Remaining proactive at all times.

These points can guide good leadership in the New Normal. Change has been turning from the initial exception into routine and so leadership needs to adapt as well — leadership has been transformed again and turns out to be even more challenging:

Leadership has to make things happen without certainty and controllable environments — a true game changer.

There are plenty of changes, adaptations, and challenges a leader in the New Normal will be exposed to. Such changes will require distinct leadership skills in order to successfully lead in the New Normal. The return on investment in good leadership and leadership skills in terms of higher organizational performance has been proven in numerous studies.

However, as leading in the New Normal is not only data driven, but, as pointed out before, concerned with the followers, another important aspect considered for leadership in the New Normal is mental health. Empathetic leaders are called for to help people navigate the abovementioned rough seas. As the Covid-19 pandemic had been progressing, mental health came more and more into the focus of discussions, as these constant and unplanned changes in behavior, the environment, and conditions proved to be very taxing for many. Mental health is a driver for satisfaction in life. This implies the necessity to be able to manage stress appropriately, both in life in general as well as on the job. Again, good leaders will need to keep in mind the aspect of stress as a driver for improving or deteriorating mental health of employees as stress can have both positive (driving performance) and negative aspects (limiting performance). This, in combination with a greater focus on work–life balance, will become a distinctive factor in leadership in the years to come. Good, empathetic, and transformational leaders will take these factors into account and make these a focus — and at the same a competitive advantage vis-à-vis their competitors.

Leading (through) Change in the New Normal requires substantial skills from the person(s) in charge. As mentioned above, authentic, empathetic, and agile leadership is needed to work and navigate through various situations successfully while remaining sharp and on point with observations, walking the talk, and acting as a role model, in order to be able to be a truly transformational leader in the New Normal.

References

[1] Beugelsdijk, S. and Welzel, C. (2018). Dimensions and dynamics of national culture: Synthesizing Hofstede with Inglehart. *Journal of Cross-Cultural Psychology*, 49(10), 1469–1505.

[2] Northouse, P. (2016). *Leadership*. Los Angeles, CA: SAGE.

[3] Kotter, J. P. (1990). *A Force for Change: How Leadership Differs from Management*. New York: Free Press.

[4] Greenleaf, R. K. (1970). *The Servant as Leader*. South Orange, NJ, Robert K. Greenleaf Publishing Center.

[5] O'Toole, J. (1995). *Leading Change: Overcoming the Ideology of Comfort and the Tyranny of Custom*. San Francisco, CA: The Jossey-Bass Management Series.

Chapter 11

Reflections on Teaching and Learning with Technology in a Pandemic-Induced eLearning Environment

Thomas Menkhoff*, Lydia Teo Ying Qian*,
Magdeleine Lew Duan Ning[†], Jayarani Tan*, and Kan Siew Ning*

*Lee Kong Chian School of Business,
Singapore Management University, Singapore
[†]Centre for Teaching Excellence,
Singapore Management University, Singapore

The Covid-19 pandemic has disrupted traditional ways of teaching and learning at institutions of higher learning. When Covid-19 hit, educators were forced to conduct classes online so that students could continue to learn from anywhere. One key pedagogical challenge was (and still is) the need to effectively design the online learning experience so that students are engaged and stay motivated. Virtual talk-and-chalk lectures are insufficient to overcome the social distance in a pandemic-induced eLearning environment. Good instructional design is critical to develop engaging assignments for learners who rely on online learning approaches and to select effective methods for imparting the desired competencies to them. The chapter reflects on the general experiences of the authors with teaching and learning with technology in a dynamic, pandemic-induced eLearning environment and outlines several recommendations for engaging and motivating online learners.

1. Introduction

Many of us can still remember Prime Minister Lee Hsien Loong's National Day Rally speech in 2004 [1] when the "Teach Less, Learn More" vision was first mentioned. Building on the Ministry of Education's "Thinking School, Learning Nation" vision (introduced in 1997 to steer Singapore's education system toward greater creativity, critical thinking, and lifelong learning), PM Lee urged educators to "teach less to our students so that they will learn more." The first author of this paper found this paradox highly inspirational as he had experienced the somehow limiting results of memorization-based study approaches of students when they first entered university and had to get used to analyzing information and giving their views in class. As Singapore continued to move from a knowledge-based economy to a creative global innovation city, the pitfalls of rote learning in terms of truly engaging our youth and making them "future-ready" had become quite obvious.

Fast forward to 2020 when the Covid-19 crisis hit Singapore, the new mantra became "Teach and Learn from Anywhere." In line with many other countries, the Singapore Government endorsed measures such as closing non-essential workplaces and suspending schools. The virtual classroom became the new normal, forcing educators to quickly master online teaching tools such as Zoom, WebEx, Google Meet, or Microsoft Teams and related features such as file sharing, screen sharing, recording, live captions, chat, breakout rooms, waiting rooms, interactivity ("raise hands"), video and audio control, interactive polls, and reports. In just a few months' time, Covid-19 forced even the most tech-resistant educator to shift gears in order to help students "learn more from home."

One "learn more from anywhere" enabler is to effectively combine both *asynchronous* (e.g., by watching pre-recorded lecture videos or lessons) and *synchronous* (e.g., through live-streamed interactive lectures) activities at a high standard. Research on distance education has provided support for both types [2–5]: Asynchronous classes enable learners to reflect and engage with instructional materials, while synchronous classes allow students to "see" their classmates and thus feel more present and connected to the instructor and their peers. Figuring out how to balance the two approaches can be time-consuming and potentially stressful because the instructor may not know whether there is full alignment between the chosen pedagogical approach and students' needs and preferences. Technical support is critical to avoid failure.

Technology-enhanced learning experts agree that synchronous sessions should not be used for lengthy lectures. "Teaching less" during a synchronous online class is sensible provided participants regard the asynchronous learning resources provided to them prior to the synchronous class interactions as motivating. Engaging and motivating learners during a synchronous session requires several skills. One basic competency is knowing what makes (online) engagement and motivation tick.

2. Engaging and Motivating Learners

Student engagement is closely linked to learning outcomes and represents an integral component of learning effectiveness [6]. Higher levels of engagement often translate into better learning outcomes, as engaged students are "good learners." Educational research has examined engagement across different educational levels and indicates that learners' levels of engagement can vary due to intrinsic factors, or learner variables such as individual motivation, and other extrinsic factors influencing the learning process, such as the involvement and quality of instructors.

Engagement is a multidimensional construct [7]. To effectively examine and measure student engagement, it is important to choose a suitable instrument such as the *Student Course Engagement Questionnaire* (SCEQ) — a 23-item measure that is easy to administer. The SCEQ captures four dimensions of engagement: *(i) skills engagement, (ii) participation/interaction, (iii) emotional engagement, and (iv) performance engagement.* We are currently using this instrument in a study to examine student engagement in the course "MGMT240 Doing Business with AI".

Motivation has been identified as a crucial factor central to student engagement and performance. We consider motivation at the process stage of Winkler and Söllner's input–process–output model [8] as one's motivation will influence and affect the learning experience during an online class. A well-researched theoretical framework for studying motivation is the Self-Determination Theory (SDT) by Ryan and Deci [9]. Intrinsic motivation refers to doing things "for their own sake" or acting as if the task is perceived to be inherently interesting or pleasant to the individual. Intrinsic motivation is associated with positive learning outcomes in formal education such as school performance and achievements. SDT posits that humans have proactive tendencies that are manifested in "learning, mastery, and connection with others". In an educational setting, basic psychological needs for autonomy, competence, and relatedness need to be met for effective learning to occur.

A useful data collection tool is the Intrinsic Motivation Inventory (IMI) which is derived from the SDT. This valid and reliable measurement instrument has been widely used to measure intrinsic motivation [10–13]. The respective sub-scales include *interest/enjoyment, perceived competence, effort/importance, pressure/tension, value/usefulness, perceived choice,* and *relatedness.*

Table 1 illustrates examples of items which can be used to measure emotional engagement and motivation in terms of value/usefulness. A student who is emotionally engaged is eager to participate in class (SCEQ), while a learner who finds an experiential, hands-on class session valuable and useful has a high motivation level (IMI).

We are currently using the IMI to examine student motivation in the course "MGMT240 Doing Business with AI".

Figure 1 illustrates the conceptual model of that study which we intend to corroborate quantitatively. Its development is based on selected learning theories and a technology-mediated learning (TML) model aimed at measuring the effects of hands-on teaching and learning activities on students' engagement and motivation as drivers of acquiring A.I.-related competencies such as the

Table 1. Sample items of SCEQ and IMI questionnaires.

SCEQ — Emotional Engagement	IMI — Value/Usefulness
• Raising my hand or answering questions during class. • Thinking about the course content during the break and after class. • Finding ways to make the class interesting to me. • Really desiring to learn the material. • Applying course materials to my life.	• I believe that the experiential chatbot workshop could be of some value to me. • I think that participating in this workshop is useful for gaining critical competencies that will be important for future work opportunities. • I think it is important to participate in this workshop as it can equip me with practical skills (like building a working chatbot) that are valued. • I would be willing to attend a similar workshop again as it has some value to me. • I think participating in this workshop could help me to acquire the skill for creating a basic chatbot. • I believe that doing this activity could be beneficial to me. • I think that the experiential chatbot workshop is an important activity.

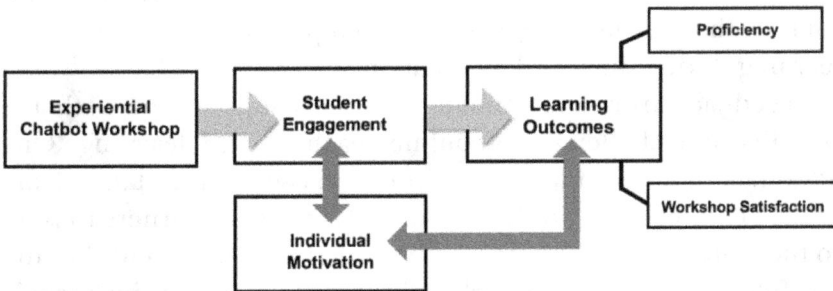

Figure 1. Conceptual model for engagement, motivation, and learning outcomes.

understanding and application of natural language processing (NLP). NLP is a subdomain of artificial intelligence that enables computers to understand and interpret human language in spoken and written form.

3. Overcoming Engagement and Motivational Challenges in an Online Environment

How to ensure that students are engaged and motivated in an online environment so that they "learn more?" A useful conceptual lens through which to approach this problem is the Theory of Transactional Distance (1997) developed by Dr. Michael G. Moore [14], Distinguished Professor Emeritus of Education at Pennsylvania State University, which refers to the perception of psychological distance between the student and his/her peers, his/her instructor/teacher, and the online learning content. The challenge is to overcome the psychological and communication gaps in the online environment through effective interaction with the learning content, the instructor, and fellow learners in order to decrease transactional distance.

To figure out how to do that well is not as easy as it sounds — even for the most experienced online educators. An ever-growing number of digital instruction tools, timely instructor training to handle unprecedented situations, technological issues such as poor internet connections, overwhelming workloads and "different types of assessments by different instructors" as experienced by students, lack of study space at home, anxiety, stress, and depression are just some of the difficulties highlighted in empirical research on online learning during the Covid-19 situation.

Feedback from our students provides support for both the benefits and challenges of online teaching and learning. One advantage is "convenience," as online classes can be taken from home. The recording of lessons makes it easy for learners to refer to the materials during revision or to catch up on content they did not fully internalize during class. Perceived disadvantages include the lack of learner autonomy and human interaction. As one of my undergraduate students put it recently, "As a people-oriented individual, it makes learning less enjoyable as I felt isolated from the rest of the class. It also makes me less willing to participate in discussions online as there is no one I know in class, as compared to making new friends during a physical class. Projects are harder because of this as well since I have to work with people whom I do not know. It is harder to concentrate at home due to the distractions present at home." The quote points to the pedagogical necessity to effectively decrease the psychological distance between students, instructor, and online learning content.

To create meaningful online learning experiences, it is imperative for educators to incorporate teaching practices that foster student engagement and increase student motivation in online teaching and learning. For the purpose of identifying and sharing best practices for engaging and motivating online learners, the authors of this chapter reflected on the general experiences with teaching and learning with technology in a pandemic-induced eLearning environment against the backdrop of supporting literature on effective student engagement and motivation. Based on this effort, we propose the following recommendations.

3.1 *Engaging students through guiding and supporting their learning from start to finish*

Student engagement being malleable through pedagogy can be influenced by what educators do to encourage student engagement in their courses. Student engagement is regarded as having three interrelated dimensions [15]: *behavioral* (concerning students' participation in course activities and compliance with rules or norms); *emotional* (student emotional reactions to activities, peers, and the teacher, and their sense of belonging to the course); and *cognitive* (psychological investment in activities to master complex knowledge, as well as their use of learning or metacognitive strategies).

To engage students enrolled in our course "Doing Business with AI", we conducted an experiential Chatbot workshop to impart NLP competencies to the participants. In doing so, we tried to foster a safe and open online learning environment for collaborative learning. Learners could ask questions and interact with the instructor or peers to respond to any topic-related questions or comments at any point during the workshop. Similarly, students were encouraged to volunteer and present their work to the class and invited to share constructive feedback in the spirit of collaborative learning. The workshop also deliberately included attention checkers for students to indicate their stage of progress during the guided demonstration, and they could make use of both the audio/video and text (chat box) functions to share their input or reach out to the instructor for help and/or feedback.

Engaging Students Through an Experiential Chatbot Workshop

The 90-minute experiential chatbot workshop was conducted online during a regular class session in Term 1 of Academic Year 2021–22. Due to the university's Covid-19 regulations, the chatbot-mediated learning was facilitated during a synchronous class session via Zoom by using a structured set of teaching and learning materials. The workshop activities were not graded to encourage inquiry-based learning and active participation. Removing any graded components was motivated by the instructor's desire to exclude extrinsic motivation factors that may exert different pressures on the learning process such as participating only for grades. An online post-workshop survey was administered to all students enrolled in the course "MGMT240 Doing Business with AI". Table 2 provides details of the study population.

Table 2.   Student demographics.

N	Gender	Year in School	Affiliated School	Major
43	23 Female	4 Year 1	0 Accountancy	8 Business Management
	20 Males	13 Year 2	43 LKCSB	13 Finance
		14 Year 3	0 Computing & IS	8 Marketing
		11 Year 4	0 Economics	5 Ops. Management
		1 Year 5	0 Law	4 Strategic Management
			0 Social Sciences	5 Others
	43	**43**	**43**	**43**

Students enrolled in this course were at different course levels (year of study) and pursued different majors as indicated in Table 2.

In an online learning environment, students may frequently feel disengaged due to the lack of social interactions. To address this issue, instructors' prompt online responsiveness (e.g., to tackle issues arising in virtual collaboration groups) would support students to perceive blended learning as being beneficial for their learning [16,17]. This finding is also mirrored in the empirical study by Anthony *et al.* [18], who reported that instructor responsiveness positively influences students' perception toward the adoption of online learning components. In another study, Heilporn and colleagues [19] examined teaching strategies to foster student engagement. They suggested online educators should strive to build trusting relationships with and between students from the beginning of the semester. This can be done through organizing ice-breaker activities to develop a sense of course belonging and swift trust, personalizing contact with students, and planning peer-sharing activities. Heilporn *et al.*'s [19] study also revealed that guiding and supporting the students from the beginning and throughout the semester, whether in a large group, in teams, or individually, fostered student engagement. Some examples of such instructor guidance and support include providing students with feedback on their learning, realigning student discussions, and reminding students of assignment deadlines and what to focus on. The effects are consistent across both online and face-to-face conditions.

3.2 *Improving student engagement through clarity in communication*

Clear communication at the beginning of the semester can reduce student anxiety and negative emotional reactions while fostering their participation in activities.

Figure 2 illustrates the communication approach chosen to balance asynchronous and synchronous approaches based on a particular course taught at Singapore Management University (SMU) entitled "Doing Business with AI" — most recently in hybrid mode, i.e., teaching students in-person while others joined in from home due to Covid-related issues. Students were informed

Dear students,

We are looking forward to our next class session on Wed., 9 March 22 at **8.30AM**. During the first part of the session, we will discuss the **Stitch Fix case** (do note the required reading below!).

At **10.15AM**, we will host a guest speaker from a Hong Kong-headquartered AI company (with offices in China, Indonesia, Japan, South Korea, Macau, Malaysia, the Philippines, Saudi Arabia, Singapore, Taiwan, Thailand, and the United Arab Emirates).

Please note the required preps as well as the session plan below.

If you feel unwell, please stay home and email us. A Zoom invitation will be sent shortly to those students who are rostered to listen in from home this week.

Asynchronous (Before) Wed., 9 March 22	**Synchronous F2F: Wednesday, 9 March 22, 8.30AM**
In preparation for the F2F session, please watch the following videos/read the compulsory Stitch Fix case on LMS:	We will discuss how Stitch Fix does business with AI based on the following questions:
Information about Katrina Lake, Founder, former CEO and Chairwoman of Stitch Fix: https://www.cnbc.com/video/2019/12/10/stitch-fix-ceo-katrina-lake-on-the-companys-growth-and-outlook.html https://www.cnbc.com/video/2021/04/13/stitch-fixs-katrine-lake-will-move-from-ceo-to-executive-chairman-on-aug-1.html	• What's the pain point that Stitch Fix addresses with its business model?
	• In what ways does technology enable a personalized clothing experience?
Stitch Fix Key Reading: Case Study AI: Stitch Fix by W. Chan Kim *et al.* (2019): A Blue Ocean Retailer in the AI World: https://hbsp.harvard.edu/tu/f8901f26	• What's the unique customer value proposition of Stitch Fix and its revenue-making logic?
Stitch Fix Is a Mixed Bag: https://www.barrons.com/articles/stitch-fix-stock-is-a-mixed-bag-analysts-say-heres-why-51638986511	• In what ways are Stitch Fix's clients and stylists supported by AI?
Video "AI Powered Facial Recognition for Computers with SenseTime": https://www.youtube.com/watch?v=wMUmPumXtpw	• How is data science woven into the fabric of Stitch Fix?
	• How can Stich Fix continue to remain competitive in view of increasing competition (e.g., from Amazon)?
	Note: The Stitch Fix case is available on LMS!
	10.15AM: Guest Presentation by Deep Learning and Computer Vision Expert

Best regards, ...

Figure 2. Email announcement about asynchronous and synchronous T&L approaches in an elective undergraduate course "Doing Business with AI" taught in hybrid mode.

about the respective subject matter 3–4 days before class via an email which also entailed the Zoom invitation.

Besides the communication approach as described in Figure 2, educators can consider dedicating one to two synchronous meetings at the start of the course to clearly explain course structure, organization, and expectations for both asynchronous and synchronous modes. Heilporn *et al.* [19] found that this clarification process at the beginning of the semester reduced student confusion and fostered student behavioral and emotional engagement, particularly in online learning environments.

In investigating activity-level student engagement (cognitive and emotional) at six blended learning courses at two different universities, Manwaring *et al.* [20] found that students' perceptions of activity importance had a strong influence on engagement. Students who rated the specific learning activities as "important to them" and reported that they could relate the material to previous learning experienced increased cognitive and emotional engagement. An implication arising from this finding is that educators should clearly communicate the value of each learning experience to facilitate student engagement, regardless of the modality (face-to-face or online) in which the learning activity occurs. Educators' general availability to address students' concerns, using video conferencing tools (e.g., Zoom) and course discussion fora to respond to students' questions, and sending regular reminders to students on course deadlines exemplify effective educator behaviors that promote good communication with students [21].

3.3 *Developing meaningful online educational experiences*

One of the most influential models in developing meaningful online educational experiences is the community of inquiry (CoI) framework (Figure 3) introduced by Garrison, Anderson, and Archer [15].

According to Garrison *et al.*, online community building has positive effects on the quality of student learning, increases student engagement, and encourages motivation of students in online

Community of Inquiry

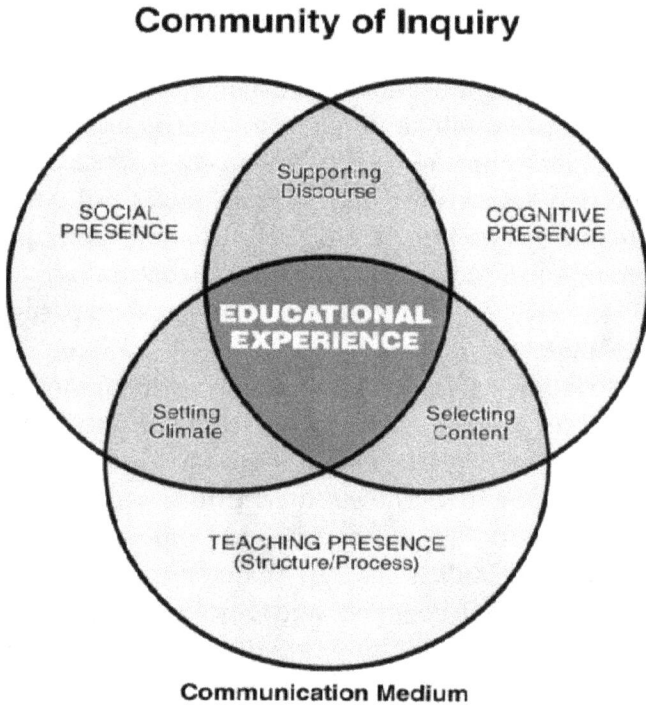

Communication Medium

Figure 3.　Elements of an educational experience [14].

courses. It is through the skillful marshaling of *social* (the ability to project one's personal identity in the online community so that she or he is perceived as a "real" person [15]), *cognitive* (the ability to construct and confirm meaning through sustained reflection [22]), and *teaching* (design, facilitation, and direction of cognitive and social processes for the purpose of realizing personally meaningful and educational worthwhile learning outcomes [22]) presences that educators can develop a productive online learning environment through which knowledge is constructed.

To help educators navigate these student online presences and harness their benefits in increasing student engagement and motivation in online learning, some ways to implement CoI instructional activities in practice are detailed in Table 3.

Table 3. Examples of instructional activities for the different CoI presences.

CoI Framework Presence	Instructional Activities
Social Presence	• Introduce ice-breaker activities at the start of the course in developing a sense of course belonging and swift trust [19,23]. • Use short videos to introduce the course and the course instructor [24]. • Include real-time communication with students through videoconferencing tools, interactive whiteboards, and virtual messaging [21]. • Personalize contact with students through one-on-one consultations and coaching sessions [19]. ***What the authors did and worked well:*** • Include valuable student participation in discussions as part of course grades. • Create a safe, inclusive environment by learning about students and helping students get to know one another through group activities and group work. • Make students work within groups but change roles among students (e.g., leader, timekeeper, checker, and questioner). • Conduct one-on-one conversations with students to check on their level of understanding.
Cognitive Presence	• Provide opportunities for higher-order learning and experiential learning to engage students [25]. • Incorporate video/audio lectures as part of the course, and have students complete readings/write position papers [24]. • Use group discussion, group brainstorming sessions, and journaling/blogging to encourage reflective observation [26]. ***What the authors did and worked well:*** • Model, support, and encourage diverse points of view in online discussions. • Use gamification to engage and motivate today's learners, and that in turn enables content mastery. • Introduce formative assessments that enhance both student's learning and instructor's teaching approaches (e.g., debating a course-related case study problem in breakout rooms). • Conduct experiential student workshops (e.g., an experiential Chatbot workshop to impart natural language processing [NLP] competencies) for higher-order learning.

(*Continued*)

Table 3. (*Continued*)

CoI Framework Presence	Instructional Activities
Teaching Presence	• Ensure instructor availability so that students are aware of instructor response time [21]. • Use collaborative group projects to have students work on topics of their own choosing that meet learning objectives of the course [25]. • Provide explicit instructions for all activities, assignments, and projects [20]. ***What the authors did and worked well:*** • Provide explicit instructions to students about the course structure (e.g., email students about course information 3–4 days prior to start of the course). • Provide frequent opportunities for interacting with students, either as a team or individually throughout the course.

Engaging students online, for example, in breakout rooms requires specific competencies. Besides technical setup skills (e.g., to assign participants to groups so that students have more voice and choice in their learning), instructors need virtual small-group facilitation skills. This includes assigning clear tasks for students to accomplish, appointing a suitable group leader to keep groups on task (asking for a volunteer might also work), assigning a timekeeper, checker, questioner, etc., personalizing learning so that participants can join a breakout room in line with their learning needs and learning style, as well as scheduled brain breaks. Gamification engages and motivates today's learners, and that in turn enables content mastery.

4. Gamification

Over the past few years, gamification has become a game changer in pedagogical institutions such as schools and higher learning institutions [27–29]. A gamification platform heightens engagement and enhances motivation while transforming learning into a process of enjoyment and fun as demonstrated by various empirical research studies on this subject matter [30]. Ab Rahman *et al.* [31] examined to what extent gamification enhances the engagement of higher education students by integrating challenges, experience points, levels, badges, and leaderboards by comparing data from both gamified and non-gamified courses. Their results suggest that gamification significantly improved students' attention to reference materials, online participation, and proactivity. Gamification also helped learners to score better.

In the field of education, gamification can be used to bring about greater commitment, achievement, and involvement in the learning process. Ekici's [32,33] systematic review of 22 articles on the use of gamification in flipped learning research suggests that adding game elements into a flipped "classroom" can lead to higher motivation, participation, and better learning performance. Moodle (a free and open-source learning management system) and Kahoot (a game-based learning platform) turned out to be the most preferred platforms used. Points, badges, and leaderboards were the most frequently used game elements. The study by Kasinathan *et al.* [34] has revealed positive effects of gamification on students' motivation and engagement compared to traditional teaching modes based on the surveyed case ($n = 24$) of an educational application called Questionify (a "smart device" developed using C# and Java language) that allows users to collect achievement points as part of their Software Engineering coursework. Respondents felt that gamification can do better in education as compared to the traditional method of teaching the students.

Sanchez, Langer, and Kaur [35] extended the theory of gamified learning by focusing on the impact of gamified quizzes on student learning. Their quasi-experimental design study of 473 university students showed that students who had completed three gamified online quizzes featuring a *wager option*, a *progress bar*, and *encouraging messages* had significantly better scores on the first test compared to students who used traditional quizzes based on a question with four response options. Study findings also suggest that higher-achieving students derived more benefits from gamification than lower-achieving students and that there is a "novelty effect" involved, implying that instructors should not use the same gamification method permanently.

4.1 *Toward a higher level of interactive connectedness in a virtual class context*

Another approach toward greater learning involvement is to urge students to turn their cameras on to create a higher level of interactive connectedness within the virtual class context. Other solutions include mastering the numerous features of video conferencing platforms and online interactive teaching and learning tools, such as interactive polls, chats, video discussion boards, Flipgrid (enables teachers to facilitate video discussions), VoiceThread (learners can use this interactive collaboration and sharing tool to create media-based online presentations), whiteboard sessions, Jitsi Meet (an open-source alternative to Zoom), and Slido (an easy-to-use Q&A and polling platform).

Slido: A Q&A and Polling Tool

Slido can be used to start a session with a fun icebreaker to lighten the mood.

Be honest, you are not turning your camera on because:

— My room is too messy
— I tried to turn it on but it does not work.
— There are too many distractions present at my home.
— I am not ready yet but will do so very soon.

Another popular way to use Slido is to find out how students feel before the presentation starts:

In one word, how would you describe your mood today?

The results are displayed in form of a word cloud (a visual display of text data).

Slido can also be used to evaluate a session via a rating poll:

How satisfied were you with the delivery of today's class session?

Scale: Highly Satisfied/Satisfied/Neither Satisfied Nor Dissatisfied/Dissatisfied/Highly Dissatisfied

---

5. Assessment

Assessing students' learning and performance in an online class requires relevant formative evaluation approaches, for example, when students debate a course-related case study problem in break-out rooms (e.g., with the help of digital whiteboarding tools) and present their results to all participants, which can be captured for later summative evaluations. Final essays, projects, or end-of-term presentations are examples of summative assessments in contrast to formative, i.e., in-process evaluations of student comprehension, learning needs, and academic progress during a program unit lesson such as one-minute essays (to answer a short question), concept maps (diagramming key words representing a particular concept), or one-on-one conversations with learners to check their level of understanding.

Although class participation is largely similar whether lessons are conducted face to face (F2F) or via Zoom, each mode has some unique features. SMU's seminar rooms have a tiered physical layout (see: https://iits.smu.edu.sg/sites/iits.smu.edu.sg/files/sr.jpg). The name tents put up by students in the physical seminar room would be nearer to the instructor for those seated in the first two rows and further away for students seated behind. This provides the instructor with a different visual perception when calling out students' names or when learners raise their hands in class to indicate that they wish to contribute to the class discussion or that they have a question to ask (i.e., students seated in front are easier to recognize and their name tents are more visible). Furthermore, depending on where the instructor is facing (left, right, or center), some raised hands may be missed. In the Zoom mode of instruction, students who wish to say something can use the Zoom raise-hand function, and Zoom would automatically put up the student's video sub-window to the top of the video window list. The instructor has an immediate visual cue on who has raised his/her hands based on the chronological ranking provided by Zoom; hence, the instructor can "see" all raised hands. In Zoom mode, remembering how many times a student has raised his/her hand for the class session is cognitively easier than doing so in the F2F classroom.

6. Conclusion

In this chapter, we reflected on teaching and learning-related issues pertaining to Covid-19 and shared some ideas about how to address those. For many students, "faceless" learning at home is not always "enjoyable" as the social distance separates them from the rest of the class. The perceived lack of social presence and exchange with "real" people can have a negative impact upon class interactions and the desired learning outcomes in an online course. To enhance "the awareness of others" and "proximity with others" (two dimensions for social presence), instructors need to master the various features of cloud-based video communications apps such as Zoom. Students must "buy into" and engage in virtual learning activities, which requires cooperating with the instructors and participating actively as per the instructional design of the online session.

Furthermore, educators must be aware of learners' vulnerabilities that could potentially affect online learning success during the pandemic ranging from monetary concerns, illness, anxiety, and loss of loved ones to unstable internet connections and lack of a suitable space to learn.

Besides cognitive "too many tools — too little time" overload, lack of bonding opportunities, lack of privacy at home, and so on, unintended knowledge loss is a real danger in a virtual classroom setting given the potential fault lines pertaining to "effective" digital information and knowledge sharing among instructor and students due to faceless (no social cues!) learning.

Many educators find it challenging to effectively combine both asynchronous and synchronous activities in a manner to enable online teaching and learning effectiveness. The inability to enumerate the necessary quantity of face-to-face and online teaching and learning further complicates the process of their instructional design.

Both inexperienced and expert instructors are well advised to revisit the basics of "good" instructional design for online learning and to consider their students' learning expectations and learning styles before they decide what actual materials and methods to develop and include in online courses to mitigate student frustration over the roll out and scheduling of asynchronous and synchronous learning components.

By considering some of our recommendations for improving student engagement and motivation in online classes put forward in this reflective article, educators can ensure that our youth will "learn (more)" in the ongoing pandemic (hopefully without getting too worried about their grades). And to all those fellow educators out there (still) coping with the new hybrid mode of teaching students in-person while others join in virtually from home due to a temporary spike in Covid-19 cases, be reminded about this old proverb: "Be not afraid of growing slowly, be afraid only of standing still."

References

[1] Lee, H. (2004). National Day Rally 2004. Prime Minister's Office Singapore. Retrieved from: https://www.pmo.gov.sg/Newsroom/prime-minister-lee-hsien-loongs-national-day-rally-2004-english. Accessed on: 23 March 2022.

[2] Chao, K.-J., Hung, I.-C., and Chen, N.-S. (2012). On the design of online synchronous assessments in a synchronous cyber classroom. *Journal of Computer Assisted Learning*, **28**(4), 379–395. https://doi.org/10.1111/j.1365-2729.2011.00463.x.

[3] Jung, Y. and Lee, J. (2018). Learning engagement and persistence in Massive Open Online Courses (MOOCS). *Computers and Education*, **122**, 9–22. https://doi.org/10.1016/j.compedu.2018.02.013.

[4] Kim, N., Cha, Y., and Kim, H. (2019). Future English learning: chatbots and artificial intelligence. *Multimedia-Assisted Language Learning*, **22**(3), 32–53. https://search.library.smu.edu.sg/permalink/65SMU_INST/1ba19kd/cdi_kiss_primary_3703643.

[5] Cook, M. (2021). Students' perceptions of interactions from instructor presence, cognitive presence, and social presence in online lessons. *International Journal of TESOL Studies*, **3**(1), 134–161. https://doi.org/10.46451/ijts.2021.03.03.

[6] Mandernach, B. J. (2015). Assessment of student engagement in higher education: A synthesis of literature and assessment tools. *International Journal of Learning, Teaching and Educational Research*, **12**(2), 1–14.

[7] Handelsman, M. M., Brigss, W. L., Sullivan, N., and Towler, A. (2005). A measure of college student course engagement. *The Journal of Educational Research,* **98**(3), 184–191.

[8] Winkler, R. and Soellner, M. (2018). Unleashing the potential of chatbots in education: A state-of-the-art analysis. *Academy of Management Proceedings,* **2018**(1), 15903. https://doi.org/10.5465/AMBPP. 2018.15903abstract.

[9] Ryan, R. and Deci, E. (2000). Self-determination theory and the facilitation of intrinsic motivation, social development, and well-deing. *The American Psychologist,* **55**, 68–78. https://doi.org/ 10.1037/0003-066X.55.1.68.

[10] Heindl, M. (2020). An extended short scale for measuring intrinsic motivation when engaged in inquiry-based learning. *Journal of Pedagogical Research,* **4**(1), 22–30. https://doi.org/10.33902/ JPR.2020057989.

[11] Leng, E. Y., Wan Ali, W. Z., Baki, R., and Mahmud, R. (2010). Stability of the Intrinsic Motivation Inventory (IMI) for the use of Malaysian Form One students in ICT literacy class. *Eurasia Journal of Mathematics, Science and Technology Education,* **6**(3), 215–226. https://doi. org/10.12973/ejmste/75241.

[12] Monteiro, V., Mata, L., and Peixoto, F. (2015). Intrinsic motivation inventory: Psychometric properties in the context of first language and mathematics learning. *Psicologia: Reflexão e Crítica,* **28**(3), 434–443. https://doi.org/10.1590/1678-7153.201528302.

[13] Navarro, O., Sanchez-Verdejo, F. J., Anguita, J. M., and Gonzalez, A. L. (2020). Motivation of university students towards the use of information and communication technologies and their relation to learning styles. *International Journal of Emerging Technologies in Learning,* **15**(15), 202–218. https://doi.org/10.3991/ijet.v15i15.14347.

[14] Moore, M. (1997). Theory of transactional distance. In D. Keegan (Ed.), *Theoretical Principles of Distance Education* (pp. 22–38). Routledge. Retrieved from: http://www.c3l.uni-oldenburg.de/cde/found/ moore93.pdf. Accessed on: 23 March 2022.

[15] Garrison, D. R., Anderson, T., and Archer, W. (2000). Critical inquiry in a text-based environment: Computer conferencing in higher education. *The Internet and Higher Education,* **2**(2–3), 87–105. https://doi. org/10.1016/S1096-7516(00)00016-6.

[16] Ghazal, S., Aldowah, H., and Umar, I. (2017). Critical factors to learning management system acceptance and satisfaction in a blended

learning environment. *Recent Trends in Information and Communication Technology* (pp. 688–698). Cham: Springer.

[17] Kim, Y. A., Rezende, L., Eadie, E., Maximillian, J., Southard, K., Elfring, L., Blowers, P., and Talanquer, V. (2021). Responsive teaching in online learning environments. *Journal of College Science Teaching*, **50**(4).

[18] Anthony Jr, B., Kamaludin, A., Romli, A., Raffei, A. F. M., Nincarean A/L Eh Phon, D., Abdullah, A., Ming, G. L., Shukor, N. A., Nordin, M. S., and Baba, S. (2019). Exploring the role of blended learning for teaching and learning effectiveness in institutions of higher learning: An empirical investigation. *Education and Information Technologies*, **24**(6), 3433–3466. https://doi.org/10.1007/s10639-019-09941-z.

[19] Heilporn, G., Lakhal, S., and Bélisle, M. (2021). An examination of teachers' strategies to foster student engagement in blended learning in higher education. *International Journal of Educational Technology in Higher Education*, **18**(1), 1–25. https://doi.org/10.1186/s41239-021-00260-3.

[20] Manwaring, K. C., Larsen, R., Graham, C. R., Henrie, C. R., and Halverson, L. R. (2017). Investigating student engagement in blended learning settings using experience sampling and structural equation modeling. *The Internet and Higher Education*, **35**, 21–33. https://doi.org/10.1016/j.iheduc.2017.06.002.

[21] Matosas-López, L., Aguado-Franco, J. C., and Gómez-Galán, J. (2019). Constructing an instrument with behavioral scales to assess teaching quality in blended learning modalities. *Journal of New Approaches in Educational Research*, **8**(2), 142–165. https://doi.org/10.7821/naer.2019.7.410.

[22] Rourke, L., Anderson, T., Garrison, D. R., and Archer, W. (2001). Assessing social presence in asynchronous, text-based computer conferencing. *Journal of Distance Education*, **14**(3), 51–70.

[23] Peacock, S. and Cowan, J. (2016). From presences to linked influences within communities of inquiry. *International Review of Research in Open and Distance Learning*, **17**(5), 267–283. Retrieved from: https://eric.ed.gov/?id=EJ1117447.

[24] Seckman, C. (2018). Impact of interactive video communication versus text-based feedback on teaching, social, and cognitive presence in online learning communities. *Nurse Educator*, **43**(1), 18–22. https://doi.org/10.1097/NNE.0000000000000448.

[25] Dunlap, J. C. and Lowenthal, P. R. (2018). Online educators' recommendations for teaching online: Crowdsourcing in action. *Open Praxis*, **10**(1), 79–89. Retrieved from: https://openpraxis.org/index.php/OpenPraxis/article/view/721/421.

[26] Dunlap, J. C., Verma, G., and Johnson, H. L. (2016). Presence + experience: A framework for the purposeful design of presence in online courses. *TechTrends*, **60**, 145–151. https://doi.org/10.1007/s11528-016-0029-4.

[27] Dichev, C. and Dicheva, D. (2017). Gamifying education: What is known, what is believed and what remains uncertain: A critical review. *International Journal of Educational Technology in Higher Education*, **14**(9). https://doi.org/10.1186/s41239-017-0042-5.

[28] Lee, J. and Hammer, J. (2011). Gamification in education: What, how and why bother? *Academic Exchange Quarterly*, **15**(2), 1–5. https://www.researchgate.net/publication/258697764_Gamification_in_Education_What_How_Why_Bother.

[29] Ortiz Rojas, M. E., Chiluiza, K., and Valcke, M. (2016). Gamification in higher education and STEM: A systematic review of literature. *8th International Conference on Education and New Learning Technologies (EDULEARN)*, pp. 6548–6558. International Academy of Technology, Education and Development (IATED). https://doi.org/10.21125/edulearn.2016.0422.

[30] Hamari, J., Kolvisto, J., and Sarsa, H. (2014). Does gamification work? — A literature review of empirical studies on gamification. *Proceedings of the 47th Hawaii International Conference on Systems Sciences*, Hawaii, USA, January 6–9.

[31] Ab Rahman, R., Ahmad, S., and Hashim, U. R. (2019). A study on gamification for higher education students' engagement towards education 4.0. In V. Piuri, V. E. Balas, S. Borah, and S. S. Syed Ahmad (Eds.), *Intelligent and Interactive Computing* (pp. 491–502). New York: Springer.

[32] Ekici, M. (2021). A systematic review of the use of gamification in flipped learning. *Education and Information Technologies*, **26**, 3327–3346. https://doi.org/10.1007/s10639-020-10394-y.

[33] Putz, L. M., Hofbauer, F., and Treiblmaier, H. (2020). Can gamification help to improve education? Findings from a longitudinal study. *Computers in Human Behavior*, **110**, 106392. https://doi.org/10.1016/j.chb.2020.106392.

[34] Kasinathan, V., Mustapha, A., Fauzi, R., and Rani, M. F. C. A. (2018). Questionify: Gamification in education. *International Journal of Integrated Engineering*, **10**(6). https://publisher.uthm.edu.my/ojs/index.php/ijie/article/view/2781.

[35] Sanchez, D. R., Langer, M., and Kaur, R. (2020). Gamification in the classroom: Examining the impact of gamified quizzes on student learning. *Computers and Education*, **144**, 1–16. https://doi.org/10.1016/j.compedu.2019.103666.

https://doi.org/10.1142/9789811255151_0012

Chapter 12

Conclusion

Linda Low and Lee Yew Haur

Singapore University of Social Sciences, Singapore

These are the four main takeaways based on the "new normal" that are described in the various chapters covering the economic, political, health, and social perspectives.

1. The "Twindemic" Scenario

With the waning number of Covid-19 cases and the lifting of travel restrictions across the world, it is indeed concerning to read about the "twindemic" scenario in Chapter 9 that spells out the difficulties of having to live with both the Covid-19 pandemic and the influenza epidemic at the same time in Southeast Asia. In fact, the influenza epidemic has received scant attention even before the Covid-19 pandemic and none at all during the pandemic as all the oxygen is sucked out by the coverage of the Covid-19 pandemic.

The possible difficulties mentioned in Chapter 9 include the following:

- the twin burdens of treating patients in the healthcare system.
- more severe symptoms for those infected with both viruses simultaneously, due to which clinical diagnosis, treatment, and patient management will be complicated.

1.1 *Influenza vaccination*

From the recommendations made in Chapter 9, the influenza vaccination for vulnerable populations like the elderly, pregnant women, and those with underlying health conditions is identified to be an important element in tackling the "twindemic." Perhaps the impact of the influenza epidemic should get some publicity and prominence, although finding the right timing might be challenging amid the general fatigue from all the Covid-19 measures. Once that is done, the need for the influenza vaccination can then be mentioned and perhaps could be made available at the current Covid-19 vaccination centers.

1.2 *Mask wearing*

Before the Covid-19 pandemic, mask wearing in public places was never practiced in Singapore even during the Severe Acute Respiratory Syndrome (SARS) outbreak in 2003. During the Covid-19 pandemic, mask wearing was not made mandatory in the beginning until there was sufficient stock of non-medical-grade ones in the hands of everyone in Singapore while ensuring that the supply of medical-grade ones going to those on the frontlines was not affected.

With the waning number of Covid-19 cases and with each household holding sufficient stocks of masks, whether they are medical-grade ones, the disposable kind, or the cloth ones, perhaps it is a good time to examine if we can adopt the mask-wearing habit in times when we are sick so that it limits the spread of the viruses, especially for those involved in the "twindemic" scenario.

2. Need for Global/Regional Cooperation

The need for global/regional cooperation in the "new normal" is mentioned in Chapter 3 when referring to the clean energy transition driven by climate change and Chapter 8 in the Covid-19 current and future outlook in Southeast Asia.

In Chapter 3, it is mentioned that as energy touches upon many aspects of the economy and society, the transition to clean energy will have many ramifications and this would need global cooperation to ensure that the ramifications are well contained and do not spark waves of bigger problems in the future.

The need for regional and global cooperation is also mentioned in Chapter 8 on the future outlook of Covid-19 in Southeast Asia, specifically on regional pandemic preparedness. The emergence of the Omicron variant from South Africa has also highlighted this need for regional and global cooperation on making sure that vaccine access is not just for the richer countries but also made available to the poorer countries like those in Africa so that the people in those countries could get vaccinated to limit the spread of the Covid-19 virus. Otherwise, the lack of vaccination in those poorer countries might see another variant emerging and that would limit the progress on the eradication of the Covid-19 pandemic.

3. China

China is the focus in Chapter 2 on the internationalization of the RMB and also in Chapter 6 on China's crisis management of the Covid-19 and SARS epidemics.

In Chapter 2, the RMB's role in international finance is found to be "underwhelming" at 2% of central bank's foreign exchange reserves compared with 60% for the USD, 20% for the EUR, and 5% for both the JPY and GBP. The chapter attributed this to the issue of convertibility which is the freedom to get and spend in RMB. This convertibility is very much curtailed and under the strict control of the Chinese government for international transactions for both residents as well as non-residents. As pointed out in the chapter, only with the removal of such controls toward a more market-oriented system with other conditions tied to assured property rights would there be any change in the internalization of the RMB. And such changes are unlikely to happen any time soon if the political situation remains the way it is.

In Chapter 6, the crisis management of the Covid-19 pandemic is compared with that of the SARS outbreak in 2003. Although differences are found in the top leader's role, the reshuffling of local officials, the participation of the military forces in the development of vaccines, and the development of relevant laws and regulations relating to the response, it still reflects that the leaders are very much in control and no change in expected in the political situation, as in the case of Chapter 2.

4. ASEAN–China Relations

As documented in Chapter 7, there is noticeable tilt toward China, especially with the Philippines and Malaysia. This is likely to continue as the Philippines elected Ferdinand Marcos Junior as the next president in the just concluded election in May 2022 as reported in Ehrlich [1]. Marcos's running mate is Rodrigo Duterte's daughter Sara Duterte-Carpio, a lawyer and former mayor of Davao City, who also won the vice-presidency with a slightly bigger vote count than Marcos. Marcos has pledged to continue Duterte's pro-China policies and time will tell if this will pan out.

Reference

[1] Ehrlich, R. S. (May 10, 2022). New Marcos era emphatically born in the Philippines. Retrieved from: https://asiatimes.com/2022/05/new-marcos-era-emphatically-born-in-the-philippines/. Accessed on: 20 June 2022.

Index

www.ingramcontent.com/pod-product-compliance
Lightning Source LLC
Chambersburg PA
CBHW050638190326
41458CB00008B/2331